# Cancer Prevention as We Age

A very short introduction from
The HealthSpan Institute

*Cancer Prevention as We Age*
*A Very Short Introduction from The HealthSpan Institute*
   ISBN: 9798865283300

   Copyright © 2023 Wellness Press



Printed in the United States of America

# Contents

# Chapter 5:
# Nutrition and Diet

# Chapter 6:
## Physical Activity and Exercise

# Chapter 7:
# Environmental and Lifestyle Factors

# Chapter 8:
## Regular Screenings and Check-ups



# Chapter 9:
## Mental and Emotional Health

# Chapter 10:
# The Power of Prevention through Genetics

# Chapter 11:
# Alternative and Complementary Therapies

# Chapter 12:
# Navigating the Healthcare System

# Chapter 13:
# Cancer Myths and Misconceptions

# Chapter 14:
# Conclusion: Embracing a Proactive Lifestyle

# Appendix A:
## Resources and Support Groups



# Appendix B:
## Recommended Readings and References



# Appendix C:
## Recipe Ideas for a Cancer-Preventing Diet

# Appendix D:
## Glossary of Terms

# Chapter 1: Introduction

## Understanding Aging and Cancer

Aging is a natural process that everyone undergoes, characterized by a myriad of biological changes that can affect almost every facet of our health. As we traverse through the phases of life, our bodies undergo cellular modifications, immune function alterations, and various genetic and epigenetic shifts. Among the diverse health challenges associated with aging, the increased susceptibility to cancer stands out prominently. Understanding the intricate relationship between aging and cancer is crucial for anyone seeking to navigate their later years with optimal health and awareness.

So, what makes aging such a dominant risk factor for cancer? At its core, cancer is a disease of the cell. It arises when cells in our body begin to grow and divide uncontrollably, forming masses known as tumors. Not all tumors are harmful; benign tumors do not invade surrounding tissues or spread to other parts of the body and are not considered cancerous. Malignant tumors, on the other hand, can invade nearby tissues and spread through the bloodstream and lymphatic system, leading to a cascade of health complications.

One of the primary reasons for the link between aging and increased cancer risk is the sheer accumulation of exposure to various risk factors over time. As we age, our cells have endured more exposure to harmful agents like UV radiation, environmental toxins, and carcinogens present in some foods and tobacco. These exposures can lead to DNA damage. While our bodies have mechanisms to repair such damage, they're not flawless. Over time, the continuous damage and imperfect repair can result in genetic mutations that may give rise to cancer.

Furthermore, the immune system, which plays a crucial role in detecting and destroying abnormal cells, becomes less efficient as we age. A weakened immune system might not always recognize and combat cancer cells as effectively as it once did, allowing these cells to proliferate.

Aging also brings about epigenetic changes, which don't alter the DNA sequence but can change how genes are expressed. Some of these shifts can either turn off tumor suppressor genes (genes that prevent cancer) or activate oncogenes (genes that can promote cancer). This dynamic further tilts the balance towards the potential development of cancer.

It's worth noting that aging, in itself, does not cause cancer. Instead, it's the biological changes and accumulated exposures that accompany aging that elevate the risk. Therefore, while it's true that we cannot stop the clock on aging, we can certainly influence many of the factors that make us vulnerable to cancer as we age.

Understanding this relationship serves a dual purpose. First, it reminds us of the significance of regular health check-ups and screenings, especially as we get older. Early detection of cancers significantly increases the chances of successful treatment. Secondly, it underscores the value of proactive health measures throughout life. By reducing exposure to known carcinogens, adopting a healthy diet, staying active, and maintaining overall wellness, we can modulate many of the risk factors that come into play.

In the chapters that follow, we'll delve deeper into the many facets of cancer prevention, exploring evidence-based strategies and recommendations tailored to different stages of life. Aging might be inevitable, but living those years with vitality, awareness, and health is very much within our grasp.

## Purpose and Goal of This Book

In an era where information is abundant, yet often contradictory, the need for accurate, clear, and actionable knowledge becomes paramount. When it concerns a matter as critical as our health, particularly in relation to cancer prevention, understanding and applying the right strategies can spell the difference between mere existence and flourishing life. With that perspective, this book was conceived. The overarching purpose of "Cancer Prevention as We Age" is to demystify the complex relationship between aging and cancer, and to provide readers with evidence-based insights and tools to navigate their advancing years with health, confidence, and vitality.

The primary goals of this book are manifold:

1. **Educate:** At the very core, this book aspires to educate its readers. Many people are aware that aging increases the risk of various ailments, including cancer. However, the underlying reasons, the science, and the multifaceted interplay of factors often remain nebulous. By laying out the facts, presenting the latest scientific findings, and debunking prevalent myths, we aim to furnish readers with a sound understanding of the subject.

2. **Empower:** Knowledge is empowering. With the right information, individuals can make proactive choices, adopt healthier lifestyles, and make informed decisions about screenings and treatments. We want our readers to feel confident in their choices and to recognize that they have a significant measure of control over their health, even in the face of the inexorable aging process.

3. **Inspire Action:** While understanding is foundational, it is the application of knowledge that brings about tangible change. Through practical recommendations, actionable tips, and a holistic approach to wellness, this book encourages readers to take charge of their health. Whether it's making dietary shifts, incorporating regular physical activity, or seeking timely medical interventions, every action can contribute to cancer prevention and overall well-being.

4. **Provide a Comprehensive Resource:** Beyond just textual knowledge, the intention is to create a holistic resource. With appendices ranging from recipes designed for a cancer-preventing diet to a glossary of terms for easy reference, the book aims to be a go-to guide that readers can turn to at different stages of their lives.

5. **Foster Community and Support:** One of the underlying themes of this book is the importance of community, emotional well-being, and support in cancer prevention and overall health. We highlight the significance of sharing knowledge, seeking support,

and building a network, emphasizing that health is not just a personal journey but often a communal one.

In essence, the goal of "Cancer Prevention as We Age" is not just to inform, but to transform. Aging is a universal journey, one that every individual must undertake. Yet, how we age, the quality of our years, and our health trajectory can be influenced by our actions. By the end of this book, we hope readers will not only be better informed about cancer prevention but will also be inspired to lead healthier, more fulfilling lives, and to share their knowledge and experiences with others.

Let us embark on this journey together, exploring, understanding, and embracing strategies that can make our later years not just longer, but richer and healthier.

# Chapter 2:
# The Basics of Cancer

## What is Cancer?

Cancer is a term that evokes deep emotion, largely because of its pervasive impact on our global community. Nearly everyone knows someone whose life has been touched by this disease, making it crucial for us to understand its nature and characteristics. But what exactly is cancer?

At the most fundamental level, cancer is a group of diseases characterized by the uncontrolled growth and spread of abnormal cells in the body. While our bodies naturally produce millions of cells in a well-regulated manner, sometimes this process goes awry. Instead of aging and dying naturally, some cells start to divide uncontrollably and form masses or lumps known as tumors.

Not all tumors, however, are cancerous. Tumors can be:

1. **Benign:** These tumors are non-cancerous. They can grow large but do not spread to other parts of the body. They are generally not life-threatening and can often be removed. Once removed, they usually don't grow back.

2. **Malignant:** These are cancerous tumors. Cells in these tumors can invade nearby tissues and organs. Additionally, malignant tumor cells can break off and travel to other parts of the body through the blood and lymph systems. This process is known as metastasis.

The origin of cancer can often be traced back to one or more genetic mutations that accrue over time. These mutations can be caused by a range of factors, including inherited genes, environmental exposures (like chemicals or radiation), and certain behaviors (such as tobacco use). While mutations are common and usually harmless, certain mutations can cause cells to begin growing and dividing in an uncontrolled manner.

Cancer can manifest in almost any part of the body, leading to the variety of cancer types we recognize today:

- **Carcinomas** are the most common type of cancer and originate in the skin or tissues that line the internal organs.
- **Sarcomas** begin in the bone, cartilage, fat, muscle, blood vessels, or other connective or supportive tissues.
- **Leukemias** are cancers that start in the blood-forming tissues like the bone marrow and result in the overproduction of abnormal blood cells.
- **Lymphomas** start in the cells of the immune system.

Understanding the complexity of cancer is further compounded by its ability to evade the body's defense mechanisms. In a healthy body, the immune system identifies and destroys abnormal cells. However, cancer cells often find ways to "hide" from the immune system or even inhibit its regular functioning, allowing them to proliferate.

It's essential to recognize that cancer is not a singular entity. Its diverse types, each with unique characteristics, growth rates, and impact on the body, make it a multifaceted disease. Some cancers grow and spread rapidly, while others develop more slowly. Similarly, some are more responsive to treatments than others.

In sum, cancer is a dynamic and complex group of diseases that can affect virtually any part of our bodies. It is a result of genetic mutations, often driven by both internal factors (like inherited mutations) and external factors (like environmental exposures). As we delve deeper into subsequent chapters, we'll explore the nuances of how cancer develops, the role of aging in its manifestation, and, most importantly, strategies to minimize its risk as we journey through life.

## How Does Cancer Develop?

To truly grasp the essence of cancer prevention, it's essential to first understand how cancer develops. At its heart, cancer is a cellular issue, a result of certain cells in the body behaving abnormally. But what triggers this abnormal behavior, and how does a single abnormal cell evolve into a potentially life-threatening tumor? Let's delve into this process.

1. **Cellular Mutations:** Every cell in our body has DNA, which is akin to a manual that dictates the cell's functions. When DNA gets damaged, it can produce mutations, which lead to changes in these instructions. While our cells have a natural mechanism to repair DNA damage, sometimes these repairs aren't perfect or don't occur at all. When this happens, cells may begin to function abnormally.

2. **Cell Growth and Division:** Normal cells grow and divide in an orderly manner to produce more cells only when the body needs them. Cancer cells, however, grow and divide without control or order, producing excess cells. Over time, these extra cells can form a mass called a tumor.

3. **Angiogenesis:** For a tumor to grow beyond a certain size, it requires a blood supply. Tumors have the ability to stimulate the growth of new blood vessels—a process called angiogenesis. These new blood vessels deliver the oxygen and nutrients the tumor needs to grow.

4. **Immune Evasion:** Our immune system is designed to recognize and destroy abnormal cells. However, cancer cells can evade the immune system by essentially "flying under the radar." They can release certain proteins that keep immune cells at bay or even manipulate immune cells to work in their favor.

5. **Metastasis:** The real danger of cancer lies in its ability to spread. Cells from malignant tumors can break away and travel to other parts of the body through the bloodstream or lymphatic system. Once these cancer cells reach a new location, they can begin to grow and form new tumors, affecting multiple organs and tissues. This process is called metastasis.

Several factors can contribute to the development of cancer:

- **External Factors:** These include tobacco, harmful chemicals, radiation, and certain infectious organisms. These factors can directly damage DNA or stimulate cells in ways that lead to cancer. Often, it's prolonged and regular exposures, like smoking over many years, that heightens the risk.

- **Internal Factors:** These include hormones, immune conditions, inherited mutations, and mutations that occur from metabolism. While some of these factors are genetically predetermined and thus cannot be changed, others, like a weakened immune system, can be influenced by lifestyle and other factors.

- **Genetic Predispositions:** Some people inherit DNA mutations from a parent that greatly increase their risk for certain types of cancer. However, having an inherited genetic mutation doesn't mean one will inevitably develop cancer, but it does increase the risk.

It's important to note that most cancers are the result of multiple factors interacting over time rather than a single cause. For instance, someone might inherit a predisposition to cancer and then get exposed to an external factor, like smoking, which triggers the disease's onset.

In essence, cancer's development is a multi-step process that evolves over time. Understanding these steps and the various factors that can expedite or hinder this progression is vital as it paves the way for effective prevention strategies, which will be the focal point of the subsequent chapters.

# The Role of Aging in Cancer Development

Aging is an inevitable, universal process that brings along numerous changes in the human body, both at the visible surface and beneath it at the cellular and molecular levels. The link between aging and an increased incidence of cancer is clear; the majority of cancers are diagnosed in older individuals. But why does aging make us more susceptible to cancer? To answer this, we need to delve into the intricacies of the aging process and its impact on our cellular functions.

1. **Accumulation of Mutations:** As cells divide and DNA replicates over the course of our lives, errors occasionally occur. While many of these errors are repaired, not all are corrected, leading to mutations. Over time, as we age, these mutations accumulate. The longer we live, the more chances our cells have to accumulate mutations, increasing the risk of developing cells with a cancerous combination of mutations.

2. **Diminished DNA Repair Mechanisms:** Our cells have mechanisms to detect and repair DNA damage. However, as we age, these mechanisms can become less efficient. The reduced capacity to repair DNA makes older cells more vulnerable to the mutations that can lead to cancer.

3. **Declining Immune System Efficiency:** A robust immune system plays a critical role in identifying and eliminating cells that have become cancerous. With aging, the immune system's efficiency can decline, making it less effective in recognizing and fighting off abnormal cells.

4. **Cellular Senescence:** As cells age, they can enter a state called senescence, where they no longer divide but still remain metabolically active. These senescent cells can secrete inflammatory and growth-stimulating factors that may promote cancer development. An accumulation of these cells over time might contribute to an aging-related increase in cancer risk.

5. **Exposure to Carcinogens:** Simply put, the longer we live, the more we are exposed to environmental factors that can cause cancer, such as tobacco, harmful radiation, and certain chemicals. Cumulative exposure over many years increases the risk of cellular changes that can lead to cancer.

6. **Epigenetic Changes:** Aging can bring about epigenetic modifications—changes in gene activity without alteration to the DNA sequence itself. Some of these changes can influence the activity of genes that control cell division, potentially leading to cancer.

7. **Hormonal Changes:** Aging is accompanied by shifts in hormone levels and functions. Hormones play a significant role in the growth and regulation of cells. Changes in hormone dynamics can lead to conditions where cells grow uncontrollably, elevating the risk of certain cancers.

It's important to underscore that aging, in and of itself, doesn't cause cancer. Instead, aging can amplify several risk factors and mechanisms that increase the likelihood of cancer's onset. Notably, even though aging is a significant risk factor, not everyone who grows old develops cancer, underscoring the interplay of genetics, environment, lifestyle, and other factors.

By understanding the role of aging in cancer development, we can better appreciate the importance of regular screenings and early detection, particularly as we advance in age. Moreover, it reinforces the need for proactive measures throughout life—like a balanced diet, regular exercise, and avoiding carcinogens—to modulate risk factors and enhance our body's natural defenses against cancer.

In subsequent chapters, we'll delve deeper into each of these aspects, offering insights and strategies to navigate aging with a keen eye on cancer prevention.

# Chapter 3:
# The Aging Process and Its Impact

## Biological Changes as We Age

Aging is a multifaceted process, with our bodies undergoing a myriad of transformations as the years roll by. While the external signs of aging, like graying hair and wrinkles, are evident to the naked eye, there's a complex orchestra of biological changes taking place beneath the surface. To truly appreciate the implications of aging on our health and wellness, it's crucial to delve into these underlying shifts. Let's explore some of the most significant biological changes that occur as we age.

1. **Cellular Aging:** Each cell in our body has a set limit to how many times it can divide—a phenomenon known as the Hayflick limit. As cells reach this limit, they undergo senescence and cease to divide. Over time, an accumulation of senescent cells can affect tissue function and lead to age-related diseases.

2. **Decreased Mitochondrial Function:** Mitochondria, often termed the "powerhouses" of our cells, produce energy. With age, the efficiency of mitochondria diminishes, which can lead to reduced cellular energy and increased vulnerability to oxidative stress.

3. **Hormonal Shifts:** Aging influences the production and regulation of various hormones. For instance, post-menopausal women experience a decrease in estrogen, which affects bone density and cardiovascular health. Similarly, men witness a gradual reduction in testosterone levels, impacting muscle mass, bone density, and other physiological processes.

4. **Genetic and Epigenetic Changes:** Over time, DNA damage can accumulate due to environmental exposures and natural cellular processes. While our cells have repair mechanisms, they're

not foolproof. This damage can lead to mutations. Additionally, epigenetic changes—alterations in gene expression without DNA sequence changes—can also play a role in aging.

5. **Deterioration of the Immune System:** Known as immunosenescence, this age-related decline in immune function results in a reduced response to infections and decreased efficacy of vaccinations. Additionally, a weakening immune system can become less adept at identifying and eliminating pre-cancerous cells, leading to an increased cancer risk.

6. **Alterations in Metabolism:** As we age, metabolic processes slow down, reducing the rate at which our bodies convert food into energy. This can lead to weight gain and increased fat storage, especially if dietary intake and physical activity aren't adjusted accordingly.

7. **Reduction in Bone Density and Muscle Mass:** Osteoporosis, a condition where bones become fragile and more susceptible to fractures, becomes more prevalent with age, especially among post-menopausal women. Muscle mass also reduces, leading to decreased strength and stamina, a condition known as sarcopenia.

8. **Cognitive Changes:** Brain structures change with age, leading to decreased volume in certain regions and affecting cognitive functions. While normal aging can result in slowed thinking and occasional memory lapses, more significant declines, such as those seen in Alzheimer's disease, are pathological and not a standard part of the aging process.

9. **Vascular Changes:** Blood vessels become less elastic with age, contributing to conditions like hypertension (high blood pressure). Furthermore, the walls of the heart thicken, and its valves can stiffen, leading to various cardiovascular issues.

10. **Reduced Skin Elasticity:** The skin loses elastin and collagen with age, leading to wrinkles, dryness, and age spots. Additionally, reduced oil production can make the skin drier and more susceptible to irritation.

Understanding these biological shifts provides valuable insights into the challenges our bodies face as we grow older. But it's crucial to remember that aging is not a deterministic decline into frailty. With proactive interventions, regular screenings, and a holistic approach to well-being, many of these changes can be modulated, mitigated, or even reversed. The subsequent chapters will delve into strategies and tools to navigate the biological challenges of aging, focusing on fostering health, vitality, and longevity.

# Aging and Immune Function

The immune system is our body's primary defense against external invaders, such as bacteria, viruses, and other pathogens, as well as against rogue cells, like cancer cells, from within. As with many of our body's systems, the immune system isn't immune to the effects of aging. This decline in immune function over time is termed "immunosenescence." Let's delve into the specifics of how aging affects immune function and the implications of these changes.

1. **Decline in T-cell Function:** T-cells are a type of white blood cell that plays a central role in immune responses. With age, the thymus, an organ that produces new T-cells, shrinks, resulting in a decreased output of these cells. Additionally, older T-cells may not respond as quickly or effectively to pathogens or vaccines.

2. **B-cell Function and Antibody Production:** B-cells are responsible for producing antibodies, proteins that recognize and neutralize foreign invaders. As we age, B-cell production declines, and there's a reduced diversity in the types of antibodies produced, making it harder for the body to defend against new infections.

3. **Innate Immunity Changes:** The innate immune system provides an immediate but non-specific defense against pathogens. Components of the innate immune system, such as natural killer (NK) cells and macrophages, may become less efficient with age, reducing the body's initial response to infections.

4. **Chronic Inflammation:** Aging is associated with a state of low-level chronic inflammation, often termed "inflammaging." This persistent inflammation can weaken immune responses and

is implicated in a range of age-related diseases, from cardiovascular ailments to neurodegenerative disorders.

5. **Reduced Response to Vaccines:** Older individuals often exhibit a diminished response to vaccinations. This reduced efficacy means they may not gain as robust or lasting immunity from vaccines compared to younger individuals. This phenomenon has been observed in flu vaccines, among others.

6. **Increased Susceptibility to Infections:** Due to the combination of factors mentioned above, older adults are more susceptible to infections. Diseases like pneumonia, influenza, and urinary tract infections can have more severe outcomes in older populations than in younger ones.

7. **Autoimmunity and Aging:** While the immune system's ability to fend off infections wanes, there seems to be an increased risk of autoimmunity—where the immune system mistakenly targets the body's own cells. Conditions like rheumatoid arthritis and lupus are examples of autoimmune disorders.

8. **Implications for Cancer:** The immune system plays a role in identifying and eliminating cancer cells. A declining immune function with age can mean that rogue cells aren't detected and destroyed as efficiently, potentially leading to an increased risk of cancer.

Understanding the changes in immune function with age is essential not just from a health perspective but also for the development of interventions. Here are a few implications and strategies:

- **Tailored Vaccines:** Research is ongoing to develop vaccines specifically tailored for older adults, taking into account their unique immune response patterns.

- **Anti-Inflammatory Interventions:** Given the role of chronic inflammation in aging, interventions that reduce inflammation—whether through diet, medication, or lifestyle changes—may benefit immune function.

- **Regular Screenings:** As the risk of infections and cancer increases with age, regular medical screenings become crucial to catch and address issues early on.

- **Lifestyle Factors:** Healthy lifestyle choices, like a balanced diet, regular exercise, stress reduction, and adequate sleep, can positively influence immune function and overall health.

In summary, while aging undoubtedly challenges our immune system, a proactive approach to health, combined with scientific advancements, can help us navigate these challenges, ensuring health and vitality in our later years.

# Genetic and Epigenetic Factors

As we traverse the journey of life, our genes and the way they express themselves hold profound significance. Both genetic and epigenetic factors are paramount in understanding the aging process and the various changes our bodies undergo over time. Distinguishing between these two helps shed light on our predispositions, our interactions with the environment, and the intricate dance of biology that determines our health and aging patterns.

## Genetics and Aging

Genes are segments of DNA that serve as the instruction manuals for producing proteins and guiding numerous bodily functions. Genetic factors in aging involve the genes inherited from our parents that can influence our longevity and predisposition to certain age-related diseases.

1. **Longevity Genes:** Some individuals seem to have a genetic advantage when it comes to longevity. Researchers have identified certain gene variants in centenarians that might confer protection against age-related diseases or promote longer life.

2. **Disease Predisposition:** Genetic mutations can increase the risk of diseases like Alzheimer's, certain cancers, and cardiovascular disorders. Genetic testing can identify some of these mutations, allowing for early interventions or lifestyle adjustments.

# Epigenetics and Aging

While genetics refers to the actual DNA sequence, epigenetics pertains to modifications that affect gene expression without changing the underlying DNA sequence. These modifications can turn genes "on" or "off," influencing how they function. Epigenetic changes accumulate over our lifespan and are influenced by environmental factors, lifestyle, and experiences.

1. **DNA Methylation:** One of the most studied epigenetic modifications, DNA methylation involves adding a methyl group to a DNA molecule. Methylation patterns change with age and can influence gene expression, playing a role in aging and age-related diseases.

2. **Histone Modification:** Histones are proteins around which DNA winds. Modifications to these histones can change the structure of DNA, influencing its accessibility and, consequently, gene expression.

3. **Non-coding RNAs:** These are RNA molecules that don't code for proteins but play roles in regulating gene expression. Changes in non-coding RNA expression patterns have been linked to aging and various diseases.

4. **Environmental Interactions:** Epigenetic changes can be driven by environmental factors like diet, exposure to toxins, stress, and smoking. For instance, a diet rich in folate can influence DNA methylation, while exposure to certain toxins can lead to epigenetic changes associated with cancer.

5. **Epigenetic Memory:** Interestingly, some epigenetic changes can be passed down to future generations. This means that exposures or experiences in one generation might influence gene expression in offspring, even if the offspring never had the same exposures.

# Implications for Health and Longevity

Understanding genetic and epigenetic factors offers potential avenues for interventions:

- **Personalized Medicine:** As we decipher the genetic predispositions individuals carry, treatments and preventive strategies can be tailored specifically to an individual's genetic makeup.

- **Epigenetic Therapies:** By targeting the epigenetic changes associated with diseases, it's possible to develop treatments that reverse or modify these changes, potentially treating the root cause of certain conditions.

- **Lifestyle and Environment:** Recognizing that epigenetic changes can be influenced by lifestyle and environment underscores the importance of a healthy diet, stress management, and reducing exposure to toxins as means to positively influence how our genes express themselves.

In essence, while our genetic code might lay down a foundational script for our health and aging, epigenetics is akin to dynamic improvisation, allowing for changes and adaptations based on experiences and exposures. Together, they weave the intricate narrative of our biological journey through life.

# Chapter 4: Cancer Prevention Strategies Across the Lifespan

## Childhood and Adolescence

Childhood and adolescence are formative periods of growth, both physically and mentally. While the immediate concern for most parents and guardians is ensuring their children lead healthy, happy lives in the present, decisions and habits formed during these early years can significantly influence health outcomes, including cancer risks, later in life. Let's explore cancer prevention strategies tailored for these pivotal life stages.

### Nutrition and Diet

**Balanced Diet:** A nutrient-rich diet that emphasizes fruits, vegetables, whole grains, and lean proteins can establish a foundation for lifelong healthy eating habits. Nutrients like fiber, antioxidants, and essential vitamins play a role in reducing cancer risks.

**Limit Sugary and Processed Foods:** High sugar intake and processed foods have been linked to obesity, which in turn is a risk factor for several types of cancer. Teaching children to make healthier food choices can have long-term benefits.

### Physical Activity

**Regular Exercise:** Encouraging children to engage in regular physical activity, whether it's playing a sport, dancing, or simply playing outside, can set the groundwork for an active lifestyle. Physical activity helps in maintaining a healthy weight, which reduces the risk of various cancers.

**Limit Screen Time:** With the rise of digital devices, children and adolescents often spend hours in sedentary activities. Setting limits and encouraging breaks can promote more physical movement and reduce associated health risks.

## Protection from Harmful Exposures

**Sun Protection:** Childhood sunburns can increase the risk of skin cancer in adulthood. Using sunscreen, wearing protective clothing, and avoiding peak sun hours can protect delicate skin from harmful UV radiation.

**Limit Exposure to Secondhand Smoke:** Children are particularly vulnerable to the harmful effects of secondhand smoke. Ensuring smoke-free environments is crucial for their respiratory health and long-term cancer risk.

## Vaccinations

**HPV Vaccine:** The Human Papillomavirus (HPV) vaccine, recommended for both boys and girls, protects against strains of HPV that can lead to cancers like cervical and throat cancer. Starting the vaccine series in early adolescence can provide protection before potential exposure.

**Hepatitis B Vaccine:** Administered in infancy and childhood, this vaccine protects against Hepatitis B virus, which can lead to liver cancer.

## Awareness and Education

**Tobacco and Alcohol:** Educating adolescents about the dangers of smoking and excessive alcohol consumption is paramount. Starting these habits at a young age can increase the risk of cancers like lung, mouth, and esophageal cancer later in life.

**Safe Sexual Practices:** Adolescents should be educated about safe sexual practices, not only to prevent sexually transmitted infections but also because certain infections can increase cancer risks.

## Healthy Mindset and Stress Management

**Mental Health:** Growing up can be stressful. Teaching children and adolescents coping mechanisms, relaxation techniques, and the importance of mental health can foster resilience and reduce the risk of adopting harmful habits like smoking or excessive drinking as coping tools.

In conclusion, the foundation for a healthy, cancer-risk-reduced future is often laid during childhood and adolescence. While no strategy offers a guarantee against cancer, adopting preventive measures during these formative years can significantly sway the odds in one's favor. Caregivers, educators, and healthcare professionals play a crucial role in imparting knowledge, modeling behavior, and providing the necessary tools to help the younger generation lead healthier, fuller lives.

# Early Adulthood

The transition from adolescence to early adulthood is marked by a series of significant life events, be it pursuing higher education, entering the workforce, forming long-term relationships, or even starting a family. This period, typically spanning the ages of 20 to 40, is when individuals establish independence and lay the groundwork for their future. Amidst these changes, it's crucial to prioritize health and employ strategies to minimize cancer risks.

## Nutrition and Diet

**Mindful Eating:** With busy schedules, there's a temptation to resort to fast food or processed meals. Cultivating mindful eating habits, where one is aware of the quality and quantity of food consumed, is vital.

**Diverse Diet:** Ensure a diet rich in diverse fruits, vegetables, whole grains, and lean proteins. Including various foods can provide a range of antioxidants and nutrients that combat cellular damage.

# Physical Activity

**Consistent Exercise:** Establishing a regular exercise routine, even if it's just 30 minutes a day, can be pivotal. Exercise not only helps in maintaining a healthy weight but also reduces the risk of cancers like breast and colon cancer.

**Break Sedentary Habits:** Many in this age group may have jobs that involve prolonged sitting. Taking short breaks, using standing desks, or incorporating short bouts of activity can counteract the risks associated with a sedentary lifestyle.

# Limiting Harmful Exposures

**Tobacco and Alcohol:** If not addressed in adolescence, early adulthood is the time to quit smoking and limit alcohol consumption. Both are significant cancer risk factors.

**Environmental Exposures:** Depending on one's occupation, there might be exposure to carcinogens. Being aware of workplace hazards and using protective equipment is crucial.

# Health Screenings

**Regular Check-ups:** Engage in annual health check-ups. While most early adults may feel invincible, regular medical evaluations can detect potential issues before they escalate.

**Specific Screenings:** Women should consider regular breast exams and Pap smears to detect changes that might indicate breast or cervical cancer. Men might consider testicular self-exams. While comprehensive screenings might come later in life, being proactive can make a difference.

# Mental Health and Well-being

**Stress Management:** This period can be fraught with challenges—career pressures, relationship dynamics, financial stress, etc. Finding healthy outlets for stress, be it through exercise, hobbies, meditation, or therapy, can mitigate health risks.

**Social Connections:** Maintaining strong social ties and relationships can have a protective effect on health. It provides emotional support and often encourages healthier habits.

## Family Planning and Health

**Safe Sexual Practices:** Continuing safe sexual practices is vital, as some sexually transmitted infections can increase cancer risks.

**Consideration for Childbearing:** For women considering pregnancy, understanding potential risks associated with delayed childbearing or hormone therapies is essential. While many women safely and healthily have children later in life, being informed is always beneficial.

## Lifestyle Choices

**Sun Protection:** The need for sun protection continues. Using sunscreens, wearing protective clothing, and avoiding tanning beds can reduce the risk of skin cancers.

**Limiting Radiation Exposure:** Be aware of radiation from medical tests or frequent flying. While occasional exposures are often deemed safe, it's essential to be informed and minimize unnecessary radiation.

In early adulthood, while immediate health concerns might take a backseat to life's numerous demands, it's a pivotal time to establish routines and habits that will pave the way for a healthier future. By taking proactive steps during these years, individuals can set themselves on a path that minimizes cancer risks and maximizes overall well-being.

# Middle Age

Middle age, often spanning from 40 to 60 years, is a time of reflection, consolidation, and, for many, a reevaluation of priorities. As individuals navigate the challenges of this life stage, which may include career peaks, parenting adolescents, or even becoming grandparents, health considerations become increasingly pertinent. Recognizing and addressing the evolving risks associated with cancer is paramount during these years.

## Nutrition and Diet

**Metabolic Changes:** With age, metabolism can slow down, leading to weight gain. Adjusting caloric intake and prioritizing nutrient-dense foods can counterbalance this.

**Antioxidant-Rich Diet:** Including foods rich in antioxidants, like berries, nuts, and dark leafy greens, can combat oxidative stress, a contributor to aging and cancer.

**Limit Red and Processed Meats:** There's evidence linking excessive consumption of red and processed meats to colorectal cancer. Opting for lean proteins, fish, and plant-based sources can reduce this risk.

## Physical Activity

**Stay Active:** While one might not have the same vigor as in youth, maintaining regular physical activity is essential. Activities like brisk walking, swimming, or yoga can be beneficial.

**Bone Health:** Weight-bearing exercises can prevent bone density loss, reducing the risk of fractures and indirectly supporting overall health.

## Health Screenings

**Regular Screenings:** Colonoscopies, mammograms, prostate-specific antigen (PSA) tests, and others become crucial in early detection of potential cancers.

**Monitor Changes:** Pay attention to changes in the body. Unexplained lumps, persistent pain, changes in skin moles, or unexplained weight loss should be discussed with a healthcare provider.

## Limiting Harmful Exposures

**Tobacco and Alcohol:** If one hasn't already, middle age is a crucial time to quit smoking and moderate alcohol intake. The cumulative effects of these habits become more pronounced with age.

**Environmental Toxins:** Be wary of prolonged exposure to harmful chemicals, whether in the workplace or at home. This includes certain cleaning agents, pesticides, or industrial chemicals.

# Mental Health and Well-being

**Mindfulness and Meditation:** Practices like meditation, deep breathing exercises, or tai chi can manage stress and have been linked to improved immune function.

**Stay Socially Connected:** Engage in community activities, maintain friendships, and cultivate new hobbies. Social engagement can bolster mental health and overall well-being.

# Hormonal Changes and Health

**Menopause and Health:** Women undergo significant hormonal changes during menopause, which can impact bone health, cardiovascular health, and more. Being informed and seeking medical advice can help navigate these changes.

**Testosterone Levels in Men:** A decrease in testosterone can lead to fatigue, reduced muscle mass, and other symptoms. Monitoring and addressing these changes is essential for men's health.

# Lifestyle Considerations

**Sun Protection:** Continue practicing sun-safe behaviors. Skin becomes thinner and more vulnerable to UV damage with age.

**Sleep Hygiene:** Prioritize good sleep. A consistent sleep schedule and a conducive sleep environment can support the body's repair mechanisms and reduce stress.

**Limit Medication Interactions:** Middle-aged individuals might be on multiple medications. Ensuring they don't interact or cause potential harm is essential.

In summary, middle age is a period of transition. While it comes with its set of challenges, it also offers an opportunity to reassess and recalibrate. By prioritizing health, staying informed, and making proactive decisions, individuals can navigate this stage with grace, reducing cancer risks and ensuring a robust foundation for the years to come.

# Senior Years

The senior years, often considered the golden years, bring with them a wealth of experiences, wisdom, and, for many, a chance to relish life's accomplishments. However, these years also present unique health challenges. With advancing age, the risk of developing various ailments, including cancer, tends to increase. By understanding and implementing tailored preventive strategies, seniors can maximize their health and quality of life during this stage.

## Nutrition and Diet

**Digestive Changes:** As we age, our digestive system can become less efficient. Opting for easily digestible, fiber-rich foods can support gut health and reduce the risk of colorectal cancers.

**Hydration:** Seniors may experience a diminished sense of thirst. Staying adequately hydrated is essential for cellular function and toxin elimination.

**Vitamin and Mineral Intake:** Ensure sufficient intake of vitamins like B12, D, and minerals like calcium, which can be lacking in older adults. These support overall health and may play roles in cancer prevention.

## Physical Activity

**Maintain Mobility:** Engaging in gentle exercises like walking, water aerobics, or tai chi can help maintain joint health, muscle tone, and cardiovascular health.

**Balance and Coordination:** Exercises that focus on balance can prevent falls, which are a significant concern for seniors. A fall can lead to complications that indirectly impact overall health.

## Health Screenings

**Frequent Check-ups:** As the risk of various ailments increases with age, regular health check-ups become even more vital.

**Cancer Screenings:** Continue with screenings such as mammograms, colonoscopies, and others. Early detection of cancers often leads to better outcomes.

**Bone Density Tests:** Osteoporosis can increase fracture risks. Regular bone density tests can help monitor bone health and prevent complications.

## Limiting Harmful Exposures

**Medication Review:** Seniors often take multiple medications. Regularly reviewing them with healthcare providers ensures they're still necessary and not interacting harmfully.

**Home Safety:** Ensure homes are free from carcinogens like radon. Using safe cleaning agents and ensuring good indoor air quality can reduce exposure to potential toxins.

## Mental Health and Well-being

**Cognitive Exercises:** Engaging in activities that challenge the mind—like puzzles, reading, or learning a new skill—can keep the brain sharp and possibly delay cognitive decline.

**Social Engagement:** Loneliness can impact health. Joining senior clubs, volunteering, or participating in community events can keep seniors socially active and mentally engaged.

**Addressing Depression:** Seniors are at risk of depression due to various life changes. Recognizing and addressing these feelings is crucial for overall well-being.

## Complementary Therapies

**Mind-body Practices:** Techniques such as meditation, deep breathing exercises, and guided imagery can reduce stress and enhance well-being.

**Natural Supplements:** Before considering any supplements, seniors should consult with their healthcare providers. Some supplements might offer health benefits, but they could also interact with medications.

# Advance Care Planning

**Discuss Wishes:** While a sensitive topic, discussing end-of-life wishes and medical preferences can ensure that individuals receive the care they desire.

**Legal Documents:** Having documents like living wills or durable power of attorney can provide clarity during challenging times.

In conclusion, the senior years, though accompanied by various health considerations, can be a fulfilling and enriching phase of life. With proactive health measures, regular screenings, and a focus on holistic well-being, seniors can not only reduce cancer risks but also enhance their overall quality of life, ensuring that their golden years truly shine.

# Chapter 5: Nutrition and Diet

## How Diet Affects Cancer Risk

Diet plays a profound role in determining our overall health, and its impact on cancer risk is becoming increasingly clear. The foods and beverages we consume influence multiple biological processes within our bodies, many of which are directly related to carcinogenesis—the formation of cancer. Let's delve into the intricate relationship between diet and cancer risk, underscoring the importance of making informed dietary choices.

### The Beneficial

Certain components of our diet have protective effects against cancer:

**Fiber:** Found in whole grains, fruits, and vegetables, dietary fiber aids digestion and may help prevent colorectal cancer. Fiber speeds up the elimination of waste, reducing the time the colon is exposed to potential carcinogens.

**Antioxidants:** Vitamins and minerals like vitamin C, vitamin E, and selenium act as antioxidants, neutralizing harmful free radicals in the body. Free radicals can damage cells and DNA, potentially leading to cancer.

**Phytochemicals:** These are naturally occurring compounds in plants. Examples include flavonoids in berries, isothiocyanates in cruciferous vegetables, and lycopene in tomatoes. Many have antioxidant properties and can inhibit cancer cell growth or formation.

### The Harmful

Conversely, other dietary elements can increase cancer risk:

**Processed Meats:** Consumption of processed meats like sausages, bacon, and deli meats has been linked to colorectal cancer. These foods often contain preservatives, like nitrates, which can form carcinogenic compounds in the body.

**Red Meat:** High consumption of red meats like beef, pork, and lamb might increase the risk of colorectal and possibly pancreatic and prostate cancers.

**Alcohol:** While moderate alcohol consumption might have cardiovascular benefits, even small amounts can increase the risk of cancers such as breast, mouth, throat, esophagus, liver, and colon.

**Sugary Foods and Beverages:** High sugar intake can lead to obesity, a significant risk factor for various cancers. Additionally, high sugar levels can promote inflammation, a potential catalyst for cancer.

## Obesity and Cancer Risk

Diet significantly impacts our weight, and there's compelling evidence linking obesity to multiple cancer types, including breast (in postmenopausal women), colon, endometrial, kidney, esophagus, and pancreatic cancers. Obesity induces a state of chronic low-level inflammation, alters hormone levels, and may lead to DNA damage—all factors that can contribute to cancer.

## Inflammatory Diet and Cancer Risk

Foods high in refined sugars, trans fats, and certain additives can promote inflammation in the body. Chronic inflammation is implicated in various health issues, including cancer. Conversely, anti-inflammatory foods, such as turmeric, berries, and fatty fish, might offer protective benefits.

## Dietary Patterns and Cancer Risk

**Mediterranean Diet:** Characterized by high consumption of fruits, vegetables, whole grains, olive oil, and fish, the Mediterranean diet has been associated with reduced cancer risks, particularly colorectal cancer.

**Western Diet:** Often high in red and processed meats, refined grains, and sugary foods and drinks, a Western dietary pattern has been linked to increased cancer risks.

**Plant-based Diets:** Vegetarian and vegan diets, rich in fruits, vegetables, and legumes, might offer protection against various cancers, given their high fiber and antioxidant content.

In conclusion, diet exerts a multifaceted influence on cancer risk, acting through various mechanisms, from DNA damage to inflammation. By making informed dietary choices—prioritizing nutrient-rich, whole foods and limiting harmful components—individuals can significantly modulate their cancer risk. While diet is just one piece of the cancer prevention puzzle, it's a component over which we have considerable control, offering a powerful tool in the quest for optimal health.

# Foods to Embrace

Cultivating a diet that supports overall health and reduces cancer risk doesn't mean resigning oneself to bland or monotonous meals. On the contrary, the foods that are most beneficial for health often bring vibrancy, flavor, and variety to our plates. Embracing these nutrient-rich foods can be a delightful journey that nourishes both the body and soul. Let's explore the foods that should take center stage in our diets.

## Vegetables

**Leafy Greens:** Kale, spinach, Swiss chard, and collard greens are packed with vitamins, minerals, and antioxidants. Their phytonutrients can combat oxidative stress, a precursor to many diseases, including cancer.

**Cruciferous Vegetables:** Broccoli, cauliflower, Brussels sprouts, and cabbage contain sulforaphane, a compound that has been shown to inhibit cancer cell growth.

**Allium Vegetables:** Garlic, onions, leeks, and chives are not only flavor powerhouses but also contain compounds that have been linked to reduced cancer risks, especially stomach and colorectal cancers.

# Fruits

**Berries:** Blueberries, strawberries, raspberries, and blackberries are antioxidant-rich and can help repair cellular damage.

**Citrus Fruits:** Oranges, lemons, grapefruits, and limes are high in vitamin C and other antioxidants, playing a role in skin health and immune function.

**Tomatoes:** Rich in lycopene, a powerful antioxidant, tomatoes have been associated with a reduced risk of prostate cancer.

# Whole Grains

**Quinoa:** A complete protein and rich in fiber, quinoa also provides essential minerals like magnesium and manganese.

**Oats:** Beyond being a heart-healthy choice, oats contain beta-glucans, which can boost the immune system.

**Brown Rice:** This whole grain offers fiber, which supports digestive health, and essential B vitamins.

# Proteins

**Fatty Fish:** Salmon, mackerel, sardines, and trout are high in omega-3 fatty acids, which have anti-inflammatory properties and might reduce cancer risk.

**Legumes:** Lentils, chickpeas, beans, and peas are excellent plant-based protein sources. They're also rich in fiber and various phytonutrients.

**Nuts and Seeds:** Walnuts, almonds, flaxseeds, and chia seeds provide healthy fats, proteins, and a range of vitamins and minerals. They also contain compounds that might protect against cancer.

# Herbs and Spices

**Turmeric:** Curcumin, the main active ingredient in turmeric, has powerful anti-inflammatory effects and is a strong antioxidant.

**Ginger:** Beyond its digestive benefits, ginger contains compounds that might inhibit cancer cell growth.

**Rosemary:** This fragrant herb contains antioxidants and might help neutralize harmful free radicals.

## Beverages

**Green Tea:** Rich in catechins, green tea has antioxidant properties and has been linked to reduced risks of several cancers.

**Water:** Staying well-hydrated supports overall health, aids in detoxification, and ensures that cells function optimally.

**Red Wine (in moderation):** Resveratrol, found in the skin of grapes, has antioxidant properties. If consumed, moderation is key.

In conclusion, embracing a diet rich in diverse, whole foods not only provides a spectrum of health benefits but also introduces a world of flavors and textures. These foods offer a medley of nutrients, each with its unique health-promoting properties, working in synergy to support well-being and reduce cancer risk. By prioritizing these foods, individuals can take proactive steps towards health, enjoying delicious meals that both satiate and nourish.

# Foods to Avoid

While a nutrient-rich diet can bolster our health defenses, certain foods and dietary patterns may do the opposite, increasing the risk of various ailments, including cancer. Recognizing and minimizing or eliminating these foods is essential for those aiming to optimize their health and reduce cancer risk. Here's a closer look at the foods best approached with caution or avoided altogether.

## Processed Meats

**Why to Avoid:** Processed meats like bacon, sausages, hot dogs, and some deli meats have been classified as Group 1 carcinogens by the World Health Organization, meaning there's sufficient evidence that they can cause cancer. These meats often contain preservatives such as nitrates that can form carcinogenic compounds in the body.

**Potential Risks:** Consuming processed meats has been particularly linked to colorectal cancer.

## Excessive Red Meat

**Why to Avoid:** While red meat can be a source of essential nutrients like iron and protein, excessive consumption might increase the risk of certain cancers.

**Potential Risks:** High intake has been associated with colorectal, pancreatic, and prostate cancers.

## Sugary Foods and Beverages

**Why to Avoid:** High sugar intake can lead to weight gain and obesity, a significant risk factor for various cancers. Moreover, chronic high blood sugar levels can promote inflammation, which is associated with cancer development.

**Potential Risks:** Beyond cancer, excessive sugar consumption is linked to type 2 diabetes, heart disease, and dental cavities.

## Trans Fats

**Why to Avoid:** Trans fats, often found in some margarines, baked goods, and fried foods, are known to be harmful to heart health. They can also promote inflammation and increase cancer risk.

**Potential Risks:** Consuming trans fats may raise the risk of colorectal and breast cancers.

## Excessive Alcohol

**Why to Avoid:** Even in moderate amounts, alcohol can increase the risk of several cancers. It can also impair the liver's ability to process and remove toxins from the body.

**Potential Risks:** Alcohol has been linked to cancers of the breast, mouth, throat, esophagus, liver, and colon.

## Charred and Overcooked Foods

**Why to Avoid:** Cooking methods that char or overcook foods, like grilling meats at high temperatures, can lead to the formation of carcinogenic compounds such as polycyclic aromatic hydrocarbons (PAHs) and heterocyclic amines (HCAs).

**Potential Risks:** These compounds have been associated with cancers of the stomach, colon, and pancreas.

## Foods Contaminated with Aflatoxins

**Why to Avoid:** Aflatoxins are toxins produced by certain molds, commonly found on improperly stored staples such as peanuts and corn.

**Potential Risks:** They have been classified as Group 1 carcinogens and are particularly associated with liver cancer.

## Excessively Salty and Pickled Foods

**Why to Avoid:** Consuming foods that are overly salty or pickled can damage the lining of the stomach and increase the risk of stomach cancer.

**Potential Risks:** High salt intake is also linked to high blood pressure and cardiovascular diseases.

In summary, while it's unrealistic and unnecessary to avoid all these foods entirely, it's beneficial to consume them with awareness and moderation. Diet is a complex interplay of choices, and the goal is balance. By reducing or eliminating the intake of foods that increase cancer risk and focusing more on nutrient-rich options, we can make significant strides in protecting our health and enhancing our overall well-being.

# The Role of Antioxidants and Phytochemicals

In the realm of nutrition and disease prevention, few terms have garnered as much attention as "antioxidants" and "phytochemicals." These naturally occurring compounds in plant-based foods have been hailed for their potential health benefits, particularly in cancer prevention. Let's delve deeper into their roles, sources, and the science behind their protective effects.

# Understanding Antioxidants

**What Are They?** Antioxidants are compounds that neutralize free radicals—unstable molecules that can damage cells, proteins, and DNA in the body. This damage, known as oxidative stress, is implicated in aging, chronic diseases, and cancer development.

**Sources:** Antioxidants are abundant in a variety of foods, especially fruits and vegetables. Vitamins C and E, selenium, and beta-carotene are some well-known antioxidants.

**Benefits:** By neutralizing free radicals, antioxidants prevent cellular damage. This can inhibit the initiation and progression of cancer and support overall health.

# The Power of Phytochemicals

**What Are They?** Phytochemicals, or plant chemicals, encompass thousands of compounds found in plants. They provide plants with color, flavor, and disease resistance. For humans, they offer a range of health benefits.

**Types and Sources:**

- **Flavonoids:** Found in berries, apples, citrus fruits, tea, and wine.

- **Carotenoids:** Present in carrots, sweet potatoes, spinach, and other vegetables.

- **Glucosinolates:** Found in cruciferous vegetables like broccoli, Brussels sprouts, and cabbage.

- **Saponins:** Present in beans and legumes.

- **Lignans:** Found in seeds, particularly flaxseeds, as well as in grains and vegetables.

**Benefits:** Beyond their antioxidant properties, phytochemicals can interfere with processes that enable cancer progression. They can protect DNA from damage, slow the growth of cancer cells, and promote their destruction. Some phytochemicals can also influence immune system activity and inhibit tumor blood vessel formation.

## Synergistic Effects

One fascinating aspect of antioxidants and phytochemicals is their synergistic interactions. This means that the combined action of these compounds can be more potent than their individual effects. For instance, the mix of phytochemicals in a whole fruit or vegetable can offer greater protective benefits than any single isolated compound.

## Real Foods Over Supplements

With the rising popularity of antioxidants and phytochemicals, many people have turned to supplements to boost their intake. However, it's essential to understand that:

**Complexity:** Whole foods offer a complex nutritional matrix that can't be replicated in pill form.

**Potential Risks:** In some cases, antioxidant supplements have not provided the anticipated protective benefits. For example, beta-carotene supplements increased lung cancer risk in smokers in certain studies. Excessive intake of isolated antioxidants can also have pro-oxidant effects, promoting oxidative stress instead of alleviating it.

**Recommendation:** Prioritizing a diet rich in diverse whole foods ensures a balanced intake of antioxidants and phytochemicals, along with other essential nutrients.

In conclusion, antioxidants and phytochemicals play crucial roles in cancer prevention and overall health maintenance. Their multifaceted benefits, from neutralizing harmful free radicals to directly inhibiting cancer processes, make them invaluable dietary components. By incorporating a colorful array of fruits, vegetables, whole grains, and legumes into our diets, we can harness the protective power of these compounds and support our health on multiple fronts.

# Hydration and Cancer Prevention

Water is often described as the elixir of life, and for a good reason. It's the most abundant compound in the human body, playing a role in virtually every physiological process. But beyond keeping us alive, can proper hydration play a part in preventing diseases, including cancer?

Let's dive into the relationship between hydration and cancer prevention.

## Why Hydration Matters

**Cellular Health:** Every cell in our body relies on water to function optimally. It aids in transporting nutrients, eliminating waste products, and maintaining the structural integrity of cells.

**Detoxification:** The kidneys rely on adequate water intake to filter out toxins from the bloodstream and excrete them in urine. By promoting this detoxifying function, proper hydration helps reduce the accumulation of harmful substances that might contribute to cancer development.

**Digestion:** Water aids digestion and helps prevent constipation. Chronic constipation can increase the risk of colorectal cancer, as prolonged exposure of the colon wall to carcinogens present in stool can be harmful.

## Dehydration and Cancer Risk

**DNA Vulnerability:** Dehydration can stress cells, making DNA more susceptible to environmental triggers that can cause mutations—a precursor to cancer.

**Concentration of Carcinogens:** Reduced water intake can lead to more concentrated urine. If any carcinogens are present, a lack of dilution can expose bladder cells to these harmful agents for more extended periods, potentially elevating bladder cancer risk.

**Chronic Inflammation:** Dehydration can cause a state of low-grade chronic inflammation, a known promoter of cancer development.

## Staying Hydrated: What's the Ideal Intake?

While the classic advice is to drink eight 8-ounce glasses of water daily (often known as the "8x8 rule"), individual needs can vary based on factors like:

- **Climate:** Hotter and more humid climates can lead to increased sweating and, consequently, higher water needs.

- **Physical Activity:** Exercise or any strenuous activity causes fluid loss that needs to be replenished.
- **Diet:** Diets rich in fruits and vegetables, which have high water content, can contribute to overall hydration.
- **Health Conditions:** Certain conditions or medications might increase or decrease fluid needs.

Instead of strictly adhering to a one-size-fits-all recommendation, it's essential to listen to one's body. Feeling thirsty is a clear sign to drink, and the color of urine can also be a helpful indicator. Light to pale yellow suggests proper hydration, while darker shades might indicate a need for increased water intake.

## Water Quality and Cancer Risk

The source and quality of drinking water can influence cancer risk. It's essential to ensure that your water source is free from:

- **Contaminants:** Pesticides, heavy metals, and industrial chemicals might be present in some water sources, increasing cancer risk.
- **Disinfection Byproducts:** Chlorination, a common water treatment method, can produce harmful byproducts linked to increased cancer risk.

If you're concerned about water quality, consider investing in a water filtration system, and periodically test your water for potential contaminants.

## In Conclusion

Hydration plays a more significant role in cancer prevention than one might initially think. While it's not a silver bullet solution, maintaining proper hydration is an essential piece of the holistic puzzle of disease prevention. By drinking adequate amounts of clean water, you can support your body's natural detoxification processes, promote cellular health, and potentially reduce cancer risk. Remember, every sip counts!

# Chapter 6: Physical Activity and Exercise

## Benefits of Regular Exercise

Exercise is often touted as one of the pillars of a healthy lifestyle. Its importance goes beyond merely aiding weight management or building muscle. Regular physical activity offers a plethora of benefits, from enhancing mood to preventing chronic diseases. In this section, we'll explore the multifaceted advantages of making exercise a regular habit.

## 1. Reduces Risk of Chronic Diseases

**Heart Health:** Regular exercise strengthens the heart, allowing it to pump blood more efficiently and improving overall cardiovascular health. It also helps lower bad cholesterol levels and increase good cholesterol, reducing the risk of heart disease.

**Cancer Prevention:** Physical activity has been linked to a lower risk of certain cancers, including breast, colon, and endometrial cancers. It aids in hormone regulation, immune function, and inflammation reduction, which can deter cancer development.

**Diabetes Management:** Exercise increases insulin sensitivity and helps manage blood sugar levels, reducing the risk of type 2 diabetes.

## 2. Supports Mental Health

**Mood Enhancement:** Physical activity stimulates the release of endorphins, neurotransmitters that act as natural painkillers and mood elevators. This can help alleviate symptoms of depression and anxiety.

**Stress Reduction:** Exercise is an effective way to manage stress, as it reduces levels of the body's stress hormones, such as adrenaline and cortisol.

**Cognitive Function:** Regular physical activity can boost cognitive function and reduce the risk of neurodegenerative diseases like Alzheimer's. It also promotes the growth of new brain cells and increases the volume of specific brain regions, enhancing memory and thinking skills.

## 3. Aids Weight Management

**Calorie Burn:** Exercise increases the body's energy expenditure, helping burn calories and assisting in weight loss and maintenance.

**Muscle Growth:** Strength training exercises promote muscle growth. Since muscle tissue burns more calories than fat tissue, increasing muscle mass can boost metabolic rate.

## 4. Boosts Immune Function

**Immune Regulation:** Moderate exercise can enhance the body's ability to ward off infections by promoting good circulation, allowing immune cells to move freely and do their job efficiently.

**Inflammation Reduction:** Chronic inflammation is a precursor to many diseases. Regular physical activity can reduce markers of inflammation, supporting overall health.

## 5. Improves Sleep Quality

**Sleep Regulation:** Exercise can help regulate the body's circadian rhythm, promoting better sleep patterns and aiding in both sleep onset and sleep quality.

**Deep Sleep:** Physical activity can increase the proportion of restorative deep sleep, allowing for better muscle recovery and cognitive function.

## 6. Promotes Bone Health

**Bone Density:** Weight-bearing exercises like walking, jogging, and resistance training can increase bone density and reduce the risk of osteoporosis.

**Joint Health:** Exercise strengthens the muscles around joints, reducing the strain on them and potentially easing symptoms of conditions like arthritis.

## 7. Enhances Skin Health

**Blood Flow:** Exercise increases blood flow, nourishing skin cells and aiding in the removal of cellular waste products. This can contribute to a youthful appearance.

**Oxidative Stress Reduction:** By boosting the body's antioxidant defenses, regular physical activity can combat oxidative stress, which can degrade the skin's collagen and cause premature aging.

## In Conclusion

The benefits of regular exercise are vast and varied, spanning across physical, mental, and emotional dimensions of health. Whether it's a brisk walk, a yoga session, or an intense workout, every bit of movement counts. As the saying goes, "If exercise could be packaged in a pill, it would be the single most widely prescribed and beneficial medicine in the nation." Embracing a physically active lifestyle is one of the most potent choices one can make for overall well-being.

# Recommended Types and Durations

Maintaining a regular exercise routine is essential for health and well-being. But with the myriad of exercise options available, how do we determine which type and for how long? Here, we'll guide you through the recommended types of physical activities and their suggested durations to maximize benefits and minimize risks.

# 1. Aerobic Exercise (Cardio)

**Definition:** Activities that increase your heart rate and breathing while using large muscle groups repeatedly and rhythmically.

**Examples:** Walking, jogging, cycling, swimming, and dancing.

**Recommendation:** For moderate-intensity activities like brisk walking, aim for at least 150 minutes per week. For more vigorous activities like running, 75 minutes per week is suggested. It's beneficial to break this down into sessions lasting at least 10 minutes each.

# 2. Strength Training (Resistance Exercise)

**Definition:** Activities that require muscle groups to work against resistance. This resistance can be from weights, resistance bands, or even one's body weight.

**Examples:** Weight lifting, push-ups, squats, and lunges.

**Recommendation:** Engage in strength training exercises for all major muscle groups at least two days per week. Ensure you allow at least one full day of rest between working the same muscle groups to facilitate recovery.

# 3. Flexibility Exercise

**Definition:** Activities that increase the length of the muscles, enhancing flexibility and joint range of motion.

**Examples:** Stretching routines, yoga, and Pilates.

**Recommendation:** Aim to incorporate flexibility exercises into your routine at least 2-3 times per week. It's especially beneficial to stretch after aerobic or strength training sessions when the muscles are warmed up.

# 4. Balance Exercises

**Definition:** Activities that enhance stability and prevent falls, especially vital for older adults.

**Examples:** Tai chi, certain yoga poses, and balance ball exercises.

**Recommendation:** Older adults, or those at risk for falls, should incorporate balance exercises into their routines 2-3 times per week.

## 5. Bone-Strengthening Exercise

**Definition:** Activities that produce a force on the bones, promoting bone density and strength.

**Examples:** Jumping jacks, high-impact aerobics, and weight-bearing exercises.

**Recommendation:** Integrate bone-strengthening exercises into your routine at least 2-3 times per week.

## Special Considerations:

**For Children:** Kids should aim for at least 60 minutes of moderate-to-vigorous physical activity every day, including aerobic, muscle-strengthening, and bone-strengthening exercises.

**For Older Adults:** In addition to the general guidelines, older adults should prioritize balance exercises and opt for activities that fit their fitness levels and any chronic conditions they might have.

**For Pregnant and Postpartum Women:** It's recommended to get at least 150 minutes of moderate-intensity aerobic activity spread throughout the week. However, always consult with a healthcare provider to ensure the activities are safe.

## In Conclusion

Exercise is a key component of a healthy lifestyle, but knowing how to balance the types and durations can optimize benefits. Remember, any amount of physical activity is better than none, so even if you can't meet the exact recommendations immediately, starting small and gradually increasing your activity levels can pave the way for a fitter, healthier future. It's crucial to choose activities that you enjoy and can sustain in the long run. After all, consistency is the key to reaping the myriad benefits of regular physical activity.

# Safety and Precautions for Older Adults

As we age, our bodies undergo various changes that can affect our ability to engage in physical activities safely. For older adults, while the benefits of regular exercise are immense, there are unique safety concerns to consider. This section outlines crucial precautions that older adults should take into account when embarking on an exercise regimen.

## 1. Consult a Healthcare Provider

**Importance:** Before beginning any exercise program, older adults should consult with their doctors, especially if they have chronic conditions, recent surgeries, or haven't been active for a while.

**Medical Clearance:** This ensures that the chosen activities are safe and beneficial. Doctors can provide tailored recommendations based on an individual's health profile.

## 2. Start Slowly

**Gradual Increase:** It's crucial for older adults to start with low-intensity exercises and gradually increase the intensity and duration. This approach helps prevent injuries and allows the body to adapt.

**Monitor Response:** Keeping track of how one's body responds after each exercise session can help in adjusting the intensity and type of activity.

## 3. Prioritize Warm-Up and Cool-Down

**Warm-Up:** Begin each session with 5-10 minutes of gentle aerobic activity, like walking or arm circles, to increase blood flow and prepare the body for more intensive exercises.

**Cool-Down:** End each session with 5-10 minutes of slower-paced activity and stretching. This aids in bringing the heart rate down gradually and improving flexibility.

# 4. Stay Hydrated

**Dehydration Risks:** Older adults are at a higher risk of dehydration due to physiological changes associated with aging and certain medications.

**Regular Intake:** Drink water before, during, and after exercise, even if not thirsty. It helps to keep a water bottle handy during workouts.

# 5. Choose Appropriate Footwear

**Support and Comfort:** Wear shoes that provide good support, cushioning, and are comfortable. This can help prevent falls and foot injuries.

**Check Condition:** Regularly inspect shoes for wear and tear, as worn-out shoes can decrease stability.

# 6. Opt for Low-Impact Activities

**Joint Protection:** Low-impact exercises, like swimming or cycling, can be gentler on the joints while still offering cardiovascular benefits.

**Strength Training:** Using resistance bands or light weights can help build muscle without putting undue stress on the joints.

# 7. Listen to Your Body

**Pain vs. Discomfort:** While some discomfort is normal, especially when starting a new activity, sharp pain is a warning sign. Stop any activity that causes pain and consult a doctor if it persists.

**Fatigue:** It's essential to differentiate between the usual tiredness post-exercise and excessive fatigue, which could indicate overexertion or an underlying health issue.

# 8. Consider Group Classes or Personal Trainers

**Guided Exercise:** Joining a group class designed for older adults or hiring a personal trainer with experience in geriatric fitness can ensure exercises are performed correctly and safely.

**Social Benefits:** Group classes also offer social interaction, which can boost motivation and overall well-being.

## 9. Address Environmental Hazards

**Clear Space:** Ensure the exercise area is free from hazards like loose rugs, wet floors, or clutter that can cause trips and falls.

**Adequate Lighting:** Exercise in well-lit areas, especially if balance exercises are involved.

## In Conclusion

Exercise is a valuable tool for enhancing health and quality of life as we age. However, for older adults, taking additional precautions can make the difference between a beneficial and a potentially harmful exercise routine. By being informed and listening to their bodies, seniors can enjoy the numerous benefits of physical activity while minimizing risks.

# Chapter 7: Environmental and Lifestyle Factors

## Tobacco and Alcohol Use

The decisions we make and the habits we form play a significant role in our overall health and well-being. Two of the most common and detrimental habits in relation to cancer risk are tobacco and alcohol use. Here, we delve into their impact and the reasons for caution.

### 1. Tobacco Use

Tobacco, primarily consumed through smoking, remains one of the leading causes of preventable deaths globally. Its links to cancer are undeniable.

**Cancer-Causing Compounds:** Tobacco smoke contains more than 7,000 chemicals, of which at least 250 are harmful, and about 70 can cause cancer. These carcinogens include benzene, polonium-210, benzopyrene, and nitrosamines.

**Multiple Cancers:** While lung cancer is the most commonly associated with smoking, tobacco use can also cause cancers of the mouth, throat, esophagus, pancreas, bladder, kidney, liver, stomach, cervix, colon, rectum, and more.

**Secondhand Smoke:** Non-smokers exposed to secondhand smoke at home or work increase their risk of developing lung cancer by 20-30%. It's not just the smoker who's at risk; those around them are too.

### 2. Alcohol Consumption

Moderate to excessive alcohol use is linked to various health issues, including a heightened risk for several types of cancer.

**Cancer Links:** Regular alcohol consumption can lead to cancers of the mouth, throat, esophagus, liver, breast, colon, and rectum. The risk increases with the amount of alcohol consumed.

**How Alcohol Promotes Cancer:** Alcohol acts as an irritant, especially in the mouth and throat. Cells damaged by the alcohol may try to repair themselves, leading to DNA changes that can be a step toward cancer. Additionally, alcohol can increase estrogen levels, which might explain its link to breast cancer.

**Alcohol and Tobacco Together:** The combined effect of drinking and smoking significantly raises the risk of cancers more than using either alone.

## 3. The "Safe" Amount

**Tobacco:** There's no safe level of tobacco use. Even "light" or "occasional" smoking can be harmful. The best action is to quit entirely, and the benefits of quitting begin immediately, regardless of how long or how much one has smoked.

**Alcohol:** If you choose to drink alcohol, do so in moderation. For women, this means up to one drink per day, and for men, up to two drinks per day. However, for cancer prevention, it's best not to drink alcohol at all.

## 4. Overcoming Addiction

**Seek Support:** Both tobacco and alcohol can be addictive, but various resources can help individuals quit. This includes counseling, medications, and support groups. It's essential to find what works best for you and seek the necessary support.

**Benefits of Quitting:** Quitting tobacco and limiting alcohol can decrease cancer risk significantly. The body begins to repair itself almost immediately after one stops smoking. Similarly, abstaining from alcohol can reduce inflammation, improve liver function, and decrease cancer risk.

# In Conclusion

While societal norms and personal choices can sometimes minimize the perceived risks associated with tobacco and alcohol use, the evidence is clear: both substances significantly increase the risk of various cancers. Awareness is the first step. Making informed decisions about consumption and seeking support when necessary can substantially impact long-term health and cancer risk. Recognizing the dangers and taking proactive steps towards a healthier lifestyle is paramount for prevention.

# UV Exposure and Skin Cancer Prevention

Ultraviolet (UV) radiation from the sun and artificial sources, such as tanning beds, has been classified as a proven human carcinogen by health organizations worldwide. While the sun offers numerous benefits, including the synthesis of vitamin D, excessive UV exposure can lead to skin damage, premature aging, and an increased risk of skin cancer. This section delves into the relationship between UV exposure and skin cancer and offers strategies for prevention.

## 1. Understanding UV Radiation

**Types of UV Rays:** There are three types of UV rays – UVA, UVB, and UVC. While UVC rays don't reach the Earth's surface, UVA and UVB rays do, with UVA rays being more prevalent and penetrating deeper into the skin.

**UV and Skin Damage:** Chronic exposure to UV rays damages the DNA in our skin cells, leading to mutations. Over time, these mutations can accumulate, leading to skin cancer.

## 2. Skin Cancer Types

**Melanoma:** The deadliest form of skin cancer, melanoma, arises in the pigment-producing cells. Early detection is crucial, as advanced melanoma can be challenging to treat.

**Non-Melanoma:** This category includes basal cell carcinoma (BCC) and squamous cell carcinoma (SCC). While less deadly than melanoma, they can still lead to disfigurement and health complications if not treated early.

## 3. Risk Factors

**Intense Sun Exposure:** Experiencing frequent sunburns, especially in childhood, can increase the risk of melanoma later in life.

**Tanning Beds:** Artificial UV radiation from tanning beds is particularly harmful and has been linked to an elevated risk of both melanoma and non-melanoma skin cancers.

**Skin Type:** Individuals with fair skin, light hair, and light eyes have a higher risk, though everyone, regardless of skin tone, can develop skin cancer.

## 4. Prevention Strategies

**Limit Direct Sun Exposure:** Avoid being outside during peak UV hours, typically between 10 am and 4 pm. If you must be outdoors, seek shade when possible.

**Wear Protective Clothing:** Long-sleeved shirts, wide-brimmed hats, and sunglasses that block both UVA and UVB rays can provide a physical barrier against UV radiation.

**Apply Sunscreen:** Use broad-spectrum sunscreen with an SPF of 30 or higher. Remember to reapply every two hours and after swimming or sweating.

**Avoid Tanning Beds:** Embrace your natural skin tone. If you desire a tanned look, consider sunless tanning products but continue to use sunscreen.

**Regular Skin Checks:** Become familiar with the moles and marks on your skin and monitor them for changes. Consult a dermatologist annually or if you notice any suspicious changes.

## 5. Vitamin D and Sun Exposure

**Balancing Act:** While sun exposure helps synthesize vitamin D, excessive UV radiation can be harmful. To ensure adequate vitamin D levels without increasing skin cancer risk, consider dietary sources like fortified foods and supplements.

## In Conclusion

UV exposure is the most preventable risk factor for skin cancer. By being sun-smart, individuals can enjoy outdoor activities while protecting their skin from harmful UV radiation. Prevention, awareness, and early detection are the cornerstones of reducing skin cancer risk. Recognizing the importance of safeguarding our skin can lead to healthier habits, a reduced risk of skin cancer, and a better quality of life.

# Household and Environmental Carcinogens

Our environment, including our homes, can contain a multitude of substances that, while often deemed harmless, may increase our risk of developing cancer. Being aware of these carcinogens and understanding how to minimize exposure is an essential step in cancer prevention. This section explores the common household and environmental carcinogens and offers guidance on how to mitigate their risks.

## 1. What Are Carcinogens?

Carcinogens are substances or agents that can cause or promote cancer. Their effect often depends on the length and intensity of exposure and an individual's genetic predisposition.

## 2. Household Carcinogens

Several everyday household items can contain chemicals or agents classified as potential carcinogens. Some common culprits include:

- **Asbestos:** Used in older homes for insulation, roofing, and flooring. When disturbed, asbestos fibers can be inhaled, leading to lung cancer and mesothelioma.

- **Formaldehyde:** Found in pressed wood products, glues, adhesives, and some insulation materials. Chronic exposure can increase the risk of nasopharyngeal cancer and leukemia.
- **Radon:** A natural radioactive gas that can enter homes through the ground. Prolonged exposure is the second leading cause of lung cancer, after smoking.

## 3. Environmental Carcinogens

Outside of the household, several environmental factors can heighten cancer risk;

- **Air Pollution:** Pollutants like benzene, formaldehyde, and polycyclic aromatic hydrocarbons (PAHs) can increase the risk of lung and other cancers.
- **Pesticides:** Some pesticides have been linked to cancers like leukemia, lymphoma, brain, kidney, and prostate cancers.
- **Heavy Metals:** Metals like arsenic, cadmium, and chromium can be found in some drinking water sources and workplaces, elevating the risk for various cancers.

## 4. Mitigating the Risks

**Test for Radon:** Radon is odorless and colorless, making testing the only way to detect its presence. If levels are high, professional mitigation can reduce the risk.

**Minimize Asbestos Exposure:** If you suspect your home contains asbestos, hire a professional for assessment and removal. Do not attempt to remove it yourself.

**Limit Chemical Exposure:** Opt for natural or green cleaning products. If using chemicals, ensure proper ventilation and wear protective gloves.

**Water Filtration:** Use water filters that can remove common contaminants, and consider periodic testing of your home's water supply.

**Stay Informed:** Familiarize yourself with the hazardous substances in your region, and stay updated with public health advisories.

## 5. Push for Regulation and Advocacy

**Regulation:** Stronger regulations can help reduce the amount of harmful chemicals in household products and the environment.

**Support Research:** Backing scientific research can lead to a better understanding of carcinogens and ways to combat their effects.

**Community Involvement:** Join or support local environmental groups to push for cleaner air and water in your community.

## In Conclusion

Our surroundings play a significant role in our health. By being aware of the potential carcinogens in our environment and homes and taking steps to minimize exposure, we can significantly reduce our cancer risk. An informed and proactive approach, combined with community involvement and advocacy, can pave the way for a healthier future.

# Stress, Sleep, and Cancer Prevention

In our fast-paced world, many people grapple with the challenges of stress and insufficient sleep. While these issues might seem merely inconvenient or uncomfortable, there's growing evidence to suggest they may also play a role in cancer risk. This section explores the interplay between stress, sleep, and cancer prevention, shedding light on why prioritizing mental well-being and restful sleep might be just as critical as diet and exercise in the battle against cancer.

## 1. The Biology of Stress

**Stress Response:** When faced with a stressor, the body releases cortisol and other stress hormones. These are essential for short-term responses, but chronic stress can lead to prolonged elevated levels, which can be detrimental.

**Chronic Stress:** Persistent stress can suppress the immune system, increase inflammation, and lead to hormonal imbalances—all of which may elevate cancer risk.

## 2. Sleep and Its Regenerative Role

**Restorative Function:** Sleep allows the body to repair at a cellular level. It plays a pivotal role in immune function, metabolic regulation, and hormonal balance.

**Sleep Disruption:** Chronic sleep deprivation can lead to immune suppression, inflammation, and an increased production of stress hormones, factors associated with elevated cancer risk.

## 3. The Stress-Sleep-Cancer Connection

**Immune Function:** Both chronic stress and lack of sleep can weaken the immune system, reducing the body's ability to fend off or destroy cancer cells.

**Hormonal Imbalance:** Stress and sleep disruption can alter hormone production, potentially promoting the growth of certain tumors.

**Inflammation:** Chronic inflammation, which can be exacerbated by stress and sleep deprivation, has been linked to several cancer types.

## 4. Reducing Stress for Cancer Prevention

**Mindfulness and Meditation:** Practices like meditation, deep breathing, and progressive muscle relaxation can combat stress, bringing both immediate relief and long-term benefits.

**Physical Activity:** Regular exercise can reduce stress hormone levels, boost mood through the release of endorphins, and improve sleep quality.

**Social Connections:** Engaging in social activities, maintaining close relationships, and seeking support can buffer against the negative effects of stress.

**Professional Counseling:** Therapists or counselors can provide coping strategies and cognitive-behavioral techniques to manage stress.

## 5. Prioritizing Sleep for Optimal Health

**Consistent Sleep Schedule:** Going to bed and waking up at the same time every day can stabilize your internal clock and improve sleep quality.

**Sleep Environment:** Ensure your bedroom is dark, quiet, and cool. Consider using blackout curtains, earplugs, or white noise machines if necessary.

**Limit Stimulants:** Avoid caffeine and nicotine close to bedtime, as they can interfere with sleep.

**Relaxation Techniques:** Incorporating calming activities, such as reading or taking a warm bath before bed, can promote better sleep.

## 6. The Bigger Picture

While it's crucial to recognize the potential links between stress, sleep, and cancer, it's equally vital to understand these are just pieces of the broader cancer prevention puzzle. Reducing stress and ensuring adequate sleep should be integrated with other preventive measures like a balanced diet, regular exercise, and routine medical checkups.

## In Conclusion

The intricate dance between stress, sleep, and health underscores the importance of holistic wellness. By addressing mental well-being and prioritizing rest, we can fortify our defenses against cancer and promote overall health. As research continues to evolve, it becomes evident that the path to cancer prevention is multi-faceted, demanding attention to both our external and internal environments.

# Chapter 8: Regular Screenings and Check-ups

## The Importance of Early Detection

Early detection of cancer can be the key difference between a treatable condition and one that poses severe health risks. Regular screenings and check-ups are paramount, not just for peace of mind but also for increasing the chances of successful treatment should cancer be diagnosed. This section emphasizes the critical role of early detection in the broader context of cancer prevention and management.

### 1. What Does Early Detection Mean?

**Definition:** Early detection refers to the identification of cancerous changes or precancerous conditions before they progress to advanced stages or before any symptoms manifest.

**Two Components:** Early detection generally consists of screening (identifying early stages of cancer in people without symptoms) and early diagnosis (recognizing the earliest signs and symptoms to facilitate timely management).

### 2. The Benefits of Early Detection

**Increased Treatment Options:** Detecting cancer early often means a broader range of treatment options become available, many of which may be less invasive and have fewer side effects.

**Higher Survival Rates:** Most forms of cancer have a significantly better prognosis when caught early. The survival rates are often higher, and the chances of complete recovery increase.

**Reduced Treatment Costs:** Early-stage cancers are typically less expensive to treat than advanced stages, leading to economic benefits at both individual and societal levels.

## 3. Common Screening Tests

**Mammography:** An X-ray of the breast, mammography is a crucial tool for early detection of breast cancer.

**Pap Smears:** This test collects cells from the cervix to detect precancerous or cancerous changes, primarily for cervical cancer.

**Colonoscopy:** A test to inspect the inner lining of the colon and rectum, crucial for the early detection of colorectal cancer.

**PSA Testing:** A blood test that measures prostate-specific antigen (PSA) levels, used to screen for prostate cancer.

## 4. The Role of Personal and Family History

**Higher Risk:** Individuals with a family history of certain cancers may have a higher risk and could benefit from earlier and more frequent screenings.

**Genetic Testing:** For those with a strong family history, genetic testing can identify mutations associated with specific cancers, informing more tailored prevention and screening strategies.

## 5. Overcoming Barriers to Early Detection

**Awareness:** Public health campaigns play a pivotal role in raising awareness about the importance of screenings.

**Access:** Ensuring that communities have access to screening facilities is crucial. This involves addressing economic, geographic, and informational barriers.

**Education:** Health care professionals play a key role in educating patients about the benefits and potential risks of different screening tests.

## 6. Balancing Benefits and Risks

Every medical test, including cancer screenings, comes with benefits and potential risks. It's essential to:

- **Understand Potential False Positives:** Sometimes tests indicate cancer when none is present, leading to unnecessary stress and interventions.
- **Be Aware of Overdiagnosis:** Detecting and treating a cancer that would not have caused harm in a person's lifetime can result in unnecessary treatments.
- **Stay Informed:** Engage in open dialogue with health care providers to understand the best screening strategies based on individual risks and the latest scientific evidence.

## In Conclusion

Early detection of cancer, facilitated by regular screenings and check-ups, is a cornerstone of effective cancer prevention and management. While there are undeniable benefits to detecting and treating cancers at an early stage, individuals should remain informed and consult with healthcare professionals to make the best decisions for their unique circumstances. As with all aspects of health, a proactive, informed, and balanced approach is key.

# Common Screenings by Age

As we traverse the journey of life, our health needs evolve, and so does the importance of different medical screenings. Cancer screenings are no exception. Based on age, risk factors, and general health, certain screenings become more pertinent. Let's delve into the typical screenings recommended across various age groups.

## 1. Young Adults (Ages 20-29)

At this stage, most cancer screenings are not routine unless there's a significant family history or other risk factors. However, some basic check-ups include:

**Skin Examinations:** Young adults should be aware of their skin and report any changes in moles or new growths to a healthcare provider.

**Testicular Exams (for men):** Monthly self-exams are recommended to identify any lumps or changes in the testicles.

- **Breast Awareness (for women):** While formal mammograms aren't typical for this age group, women should be familiar with the normal state of their breasts and report any changes.

## 2. Adults (Ages 30-49)

**Pap Smears:** Women should have regular cervical cancer screenings starting at age 21. From 30 to 65, it's recommended to have a Pap smear every three years or co-testing with a Pap smear and HPV test every five years.

**Mammograms:** Depending on family history, some women might start mammography in their 40s.

**Colon Cancer Screenings:** Individuals with a strong family history of colorectal cancer or certain conditions like inflammatory bowel disease might begin screenings before age 50.

## 3. Middle-aged Adults (Ages 50-64)

This age group sees an uptick in routine screenings:

**Mammograms:** Women should have mammograms every one to two years.

**Colonoscopy:** Starting at age 50 (or earlier based on risk), individuals should begin routine colon cancer screenings. Colonoscopies are typically repeated every ten years if no polyps are found.

**Lung Cancer Screenings:** Current or former smokers aged 50-80 who have a 20 pack-year smoking history and currently smoke or have quit within the past 15 years should consider annual screenings with low-dose computed tomography (LDCT).

**Prostate Cancer Screenings (for men):** Men should discuss the benefits and risks of prostate-specific antigen (PSA) testing with their doctors.

## 4. Seniors (Ages 65 and Older)

Continued screenings remain vital in senior years, but frequency and types might change based on health status and past results.

**Bone Density Scan:** While not a cancer screening, women might be advised to check for osteoporosis starting in their mid-60s, especially if there's a family history.

**Colonoscopy:** Continuation or initiation, based on previous screenings and findings.

**Lung Cancer Screenings:** As with the younger age bracket, high-risk individuals should continue annual LDCT screenings.

**Prostate Cancer Screenings (for men):** Ongoing discussions with healthcare providers are crucial, especially if previous tests indicated potential concerns.

## 5. Beyond Age-Based Screenings

It's essential to remember that individual risk factors—including family history, genetic predispositions, and certain health conditions—might necessitate different screening schedules. Always consult with healthcare professionals to tailor screenings to personal health profiles.

## In Conclusion

While age serves as a guideline for certain cancer screenings, individual circumstances play a decisive role in determining the most beneficial and timely interventions. Staying informed, having open dialogues with healthcare providers, and proactively participating in recommended screenings can make a substantial difference in early detection and successful cancer management.

# Understanding and Interpreting Results

When it comes to cancer screenings, receiving the results is often a source of anxiety. Whether the news is positive or negative, understanding the meaning and implications of these findings is paramount. This section aims to guide readers through the nuances of interpreting screening results, helping transform medical jargon into actionable knowledge.

## 1. Basic Terminology

**Negative or Normal:** This means no signs of the disease were found. It's a good outcome, but it's important to continue regular screenings as recommended.

**Positive:** A positive result indicates that the test found something abnormal. This doesn't necessarily mean cancer is present; further tests are often required.

**False Positive:** The test indicates a problem when there is none. While relief follows, the initial news can be distressing.

**False Negative:** The test appears normal even though cancer is present. This underscores the importance of regular screenings and being attentive to body changes.

## 2. What if it's Positive?

A positive result typically leads to more tests to confirm or rule out cancer:

**Biopsy:** A sample of cells or tissue is taken from the area that looks suspicious and studied under a microscope.

**Diagnostic Tests:** These might include more detailed X-rays, MRIs, or other imaging.

Remember, a positive screening doesn't necessarily mean cancer. It could be benign (non-cancerous) growths, other diseases, or even just false alarms.

## 3. The Role of Second Opinions

If faced with a diagnosis, seeking a second opinion can be invaluable:

**Confirming Diagnosis:** A fresh set of eyes can confirm the initial findings, ensuring the diagnosis's accuracy.

**Evaluating Treatment Options:** Different specialists might recommend varying treatment strategies.

## 4. Grading and Staging

If a biopsy confirms cancer, the diagnosis usually includes its grade and stage:

**Grading:** This describes how much cancer cells resemble normal cells. A lower grade indicates a slower-growing cancer, while a higher grade suggests a faster-growing one.

**Staging:** This defines the extent of the cancer. It considers the tumor size, if it has spread to nearby tissues, or if it's reached other parts of the body. Stages range from 0 (in situ, or localized) to IV (advanced).

## 5. Recurrence and Remission

For individuals previously treated for cancer, specific terms denote the disease's status:

- **Recurrence:** This means the cancer has returned after treatment. It can be local (in the same place) or distant (spread to other parts of the body).
- **Remission:** This doesn't necessarily mean the cancer is cured, but it's under control and diminished. Complete remission implies no detectable traces of the disease, while partial means the cancer has reduced but is still present.

## 6. Beyond the Clinical Aspects

While understanding the medical facets of screening results is vital, it's equally crucial to recognize and manage the emotional toll:

- **Emotional Preparedness:** Receiving results, especially if unexpected, can be overwhelming. It's essential to have emotional support, whether from family, friends, or support groups.
- **Communication:** Engage openly with healthcare providers, asking questions to understand the findings and their implications fully.

## In Conclusion

Interpreting the results of cancer screenings goes beyond understanding medical terms. It involves an intricate interplay of knowledge, emotional management, proactive communication, and informed decision-making. Knowledge is empowerment, and understanding screening results can pave the way for informed decisions, whether they involve further tests, treatments, or simple relief.

# Chapter 9: Mental and Emotional Health

## Psychological Stress and Cancer Risk

The intricate interplay between our mental and physical well-being has been a subject of research and fascination for decades. While stress is a natural part of life, chronic psychological stress can have significant repercussions on our overall health. But what about its relationship with cancer? Let's explore the current understanding of how psychological stress might influence cancer risk and progression.

### 1. The Biological Mechanisms

While stress itself is not a direct cause of cancer, the biological responses it triggers can potentially influence the development and progression of cancer:

- **Stress Hormones:** Chronic stress leads to prolonged release of stress hormones like cortisol and adrenaline. High levels of these hormones can suppress the immune system and promote tumor growth and spread.
- **DNA Repair:** There's evidence to suggest that stress might impair the body's capability to repair DNA damage, potentially leading to cancerous mutations.

### 2. Stress-induced Behaviors

The way people cope with stress can indirectly increase cancer risk:

- **Unhealthy Lifestyle Choices:** Some individuals resort to smoking, excessive alcohol consumption, or overeating as ways to manage stress—all of which are known risk factors for various cancers.
- **Physical Inactivity:** Chronic stress can lead to fatigue or feelings

of defeat, reducing the motivation to exercise—a key factor in cancer prevention.

## 3. Effects on Cancer Progression

For those already diagnosed with cancer, stress might affect its progression:

- **Immune System Impact:** Chronic stress can weaken the immune system, potentially aiding the growth and spread of tumors.
- **Treatment Adherence:** High stress levels can impact a patient's ability to follow treatment plans, attend appointments, or manage medication schedules, affecting treatment outcomes.

## 4. Mental Well-being After Diagnosis

A cancer diagnosis is inherently stressful. Patients often grapple with:

- **Uncertainty and Fear:** Concerns about the future, treatment outcomes, and potential recurrence can be significant sources of stress.
- **Treatment Side Effects:** Physical changes, pain, fatigue, and other side effects can contribute to emotional and psychological distress.

Support from healthcare teams, therapists, and support groups can be crucial in navigating these challenges.

## 5. Reducing Stress: Strategies and Benefits

While eliminating stress entirely is unrealistic, managing it effectively can have potential health benefits:

- **Mindfulness and Meditation:** These practices can help individuals become more aware of their reactions to stress and develop healthier coping mechanisms.
- **Physical Activity:** Exercise is a proven stress-reliever. It releases endorphins, reduces stress hormones, and can help maintain a healthy weight.

- **Social Support:** Engaging with supportive family, friends, or support groups can alleviate feelings of isolation and provide avenues to discuss and manage stressors.
- **Professional Therapy:** For those grappling with significant distress, therapists and counselors can provide tools and strategies to cope.

## 6. In Perspective: Stress and Overall Health

While the direct link between stress and cancer is still being explored, it's evident that chronic psychological stress can have wide-ranging implications on overall health—from cardiovascular diseases to weakened immune function. Prioritizing mental health and stress management, therefore, is not just about reducing cancer risk but about promoting holistic well-being.

## In Conclusion

The relationship between psychological stress and cancer is complex and multifaceted. While stress might not directly cause cancer, its biological effects and the behaviors it prompts can influence cancer risk and progression. Recognizing the importance of mental and emotional health, adopting stress-reducing strategies, and seeking support when needed can play a pivotal role in cancer prevention and care.

# Maintaining Mental Agility

In the same way that physical fitness is vital for our bodies, mental agility is crucial for our minds, especially as we age. Just as muscles weaken without regular exercise, cognitive functions can decline if not consistently stimulated. Fortunately, there are numerous ways to keep our minds sharp, ensuring that we continue to think, learn, and remember efficiently as we grow older.

## 1. Defining Mental Agility

Mental agility refers to the mind's capacity to think quickly, grasp new ideas, and integrate various forms of information seamlessly. It's about:

- **Adaptability:** The ability to adjust to new situations or changes in the environment.
- **Cognitive Flexibility:** Switching between different tasks or thoughts with ease.
- **Problem-solving:** Finding solutions to challenges efficiently and creatively.

## 2. The Brain's Plasticity

Contrary to older beliefs that the brain becomes rigid with age, research shows that the brain retains plasticity throughout life:

- **Neurogenesis:** Even in adulthood, the brain can produce new neurons, particularly in the hippocampus, a region vital for memory and learning.
- **Synaptic Plasticity:** The connections between neurons, or synapses, can strengthen or weaken over time, depending on their usage.

Thus, engaging in mental exercises can indeed reshape and enhance brain function.

## 3. Mental Workouts to Boost Agility

Just as physical workouts bolster the body, mental exercises can enhance cognitive function:

- **Puzzles and Games:** Crosswords, Sudoku, and strategy games like chess or Go stimulate various parts of the brain.
- **Learning a New Skill:** Whether it's a musical instrument, a new language, or a craft, acquiring new skills keeps the brain active and challenged.
- **Reading:** Regularly diving into books, articles, or even poetry can expand vocabulary, improve comprehension, and stimulate imagination.

## 4. The Role of Physical Activity

Physical health and mental health are intertwined:

- **Increased Blood Flow:** Physical activity boosts blood flow, ensuring the brain receives a steady supply of oxygen and nutrients.
- **Neurotransmitters:** Exercise helps release neurotransmitters like serotonin and dopamine, which play roles in mood regulation, motivation, and alertness.
- **Reduction of Stress:** Regular physical activity can reduce stress levels, which, if chronic, can impair cognitive functions.

## 5. Social Engagement and Mental Agility

Interpersonal interactions can provide cognitive stimulation:

- **Varied Conversations:** Engaging with people exposes us to new ideas, perspectives, and information.
- **Emotional Processing:** Navigating social scenarios requires interpreting emotions, understanding social cues, and responding appropriately—excellent exercises for the brain.

## 6. Nutrition and Hydration

The brain thrives on a balanced diet:

- **Omega-3 Fatty Acids:** Found in fish, flaxseeds, and walnuts, these support brain health and cognitive functions.
- **Antioxidants:** Berries, nuts, and dark chocolate contain compounds that can protect brain cells from damage.
- **Water:** Staying hydrated supports overall brain health and function. Even mild dehydration can impair concentration and cognitive abilities.

## 7. Lifelong Learning and Curiosity

Maintaining a curious mindset and a love for learning can do wonders:

- **Continuous Education:** Attend workshops, take courses, or engage in webinars to always keep learning.
- **Travel:** Experiencing new cultures and environments can challenge the brain and expand one's horizons.

## In Conclusion

Maintaining mental agility as we age requires a multi-faceted approach, combining mental exercises, physical activity, social engagement, and proper nutrition. Just as one might develop a regimen to maintain physical fitness, building daily habits to nurture the mind can ensure it remains sharp, adaptable, and resilient for years to come.

# Support Systems and Community

Human beings, as inherently social creatures, thrive on connections and relationships. The networks of people we turn to for emotional, informational, and practical assistance—our support systems—are fundamental pillars of our mental and emotional health. Especially as we navigate the challenges of aging and potential health concerns, having a robust support system and being part of a community can make all the difference.

## 1. Defining Support Systems

A support system isn't just the people you're closest to; it's a web of relationships that provide various forms of aid:

- **Emotional Support:** Those we turn to for understanding, empathy, or simply a listening ear.
- **Informational Support:** Individuals who offer advice, guidance, or share their knowledge and experiences.
- **Tangible Support:** Help with practical matters, such as transportation, chores, or financial assistance.
- **Companionship:** People we share activities, hobbies, or simple social interactions with.

## 2. The Impact of Support on Well-being

Support systems and community engagements are more than just feel-good elements of life; they have tangible benefits:

- **Reduced Stress:** Social connections can act as buffers against life's stressors, reducing feelings of isolation and despair.

- **Better Mental Health Outcomes:** Numerous studies have shown that individuals with strong support systems tend to have lower rates of depression, anxiety, and other mental health challenges.
- **Improved Physical Health:** Social engagement has been linked to lower blood pressure, better immune function, and even longer life spans.

## 3. Building and Maintaining Support Systems

As life evolves, so do our relationships. But with intent, one can maintain and even grow their support network:

- **Staying Active in Communities:** This could be religious groups, hobby clubs, or neighborhood associations. Regular participation can foster connections.
- **Reaching Out:** Taking the initiative, even with a simple call or message, can maintain and strengthen bonds.
- **Being Open to New Relationships:** Every interaction has the potential to turn into a supportive relationship. Be it at a class, workshop, or park, being open can lead to meaningful connections.

## 4. The Role of Digital Communities

In the age of the internet, support and community are not limited by geography:

- **Online Support Groups:** These can be especially beneficial for individuals with specific health concerns or challenges, offering a platform to share, learn, and connect.
- **Virtual Workshops and Webinars:** Online platforms offer opportunities to learn new skills and meet people with similar interests.
- **Social Media:** Used mindfully, platforms like Facebook, Twitter, or Instagram can help maintain connections and foster new ones.

## 5. Navigating Changes in Support Systems

As we age, there can be shifts in our support networks:

- **Loss:** Grieving lost loved ones is a challenging part of life. Seeking support through grief counseling or bereavement groups can be helpful.

- **Relocation:** Moving to new places can disrupt established support systems. Making an effort to engage in local communities can bridge this gap.

## 6. Being a Pillar for Others

While seeking support is essential, offering it is equally beneficial:

- **Volunteering:** Giving time to causes or organizations can provide a sense of purpose and establish new connections.

- **Mentorship:** Sharing experiences and guiding younger individuals can be a fulfilling way to give back and form bonds.

## In Conclusion

The adage "no man is an island" holds profound truth. Our well-being is deeply intertwined with the quality and nature of our relationships. Investing time and energy in building, maintaining, and cherishing our support systems and communities can lay the foundation for a mentally and emotionally enriching life, no matter our age.

# Chapter 10:
# The Power of Prevention through Genetics

## Understanding Genetic Predispositions

The rapidly evolving field of genetics offers both promises and challenges in understanding diseases, including cancer. One of the most discussed aspects of this science is the concept of genetic predispositions. These predispositions, or genetic susceptibilities, can inform an individual's likelihood of developing specific diseases.

## 1. What is a Genetic Predisposition?

A genetic predisposition results from specific genetic variations that are passed from parents to offspring. These variations contribute to an individual's chance of developing a particular disease:

- **Genes and DNA:** Genes are segments of DNA that instruct the body how to create proteins, which in turn determine the body's structures and functions.
- **Variations or Mutations:** Sometimes, there are changes or mistakes in DNA. Some of these changes might increase the risk of certain diseases.

## 2. Predispositions and Cancer

While several factors, including lifestyle and environment, play a role in cancer development, genetic mutations can be significant predictors:

- **High-Penetrance Mutations:** These are genetic changes that considerably increase the risk of cancer. Examples include mutations in the BRCA1 or BRCA2 genes, linked to breast and ovarian cancer.

- **Low-Penetrance Mutations:** These increase cancer risk only slightly but might be common in the general population.

## 3. Testing for Genetic Predispositions

Genetic tests are available to detect many of the mutations associated with a higher risk of certain cancers:

- **Purpose:** To identify individuals who might benefit from more intensive surveillance or preventive measures.
- **Procedure:** Typically involves taking a blood or saliva sample.
- **Results Interpretation:** A healthcare professional or genetic counselor can help understand the implications of test results.

## 4. Implications of Knowing One's Predisposition

Discovering that one has a genetic predisposition can have profound implications:

- **Proactive Monitoring:** Enables closer and more regular screenings, leading to early detection and potentially better outcomes.
- **Preventive Measures:** Individuals might choose interventions, like surgery or medications, to reduce the risk.
- **Psychological Impact:** Knowledge can bring a sense of empowerment but also anxiety or fear. Support and counseling can help navigate these emotions.

## 5. Limitations and Considerations

Understanding genetic predispositions is powerful, but it's essential to recognize its limits:

- **Not a Destiny:** Having a predisposition does not guarantee the development of cancer; it merely indicates an increased risk.
- **False Security:** Not having a known predisposition does not mean one is immune to cancer.
- **Ethical Concerns:** There are potential implications for insurance, employment, and privacy.

## 6. Importance of Genetic Counseling

Given the complexities and nuances, genetic counseling is invaluable:

- **What Counselors Do:** Help individuals understand their risks, interpret test results, and guide through potential next steps.
- **Emotional Support:** Address the emotional and psychological aspects of genetic testing and its results.

## 7. The Broader Picture

While genes play a critical role, it's essential to view them as part of a broader picture:

- **Lifestyle Choices:** Diet, exercise, and exposure to certain environmental factors can influence cancer risk.
- **Regular Screenings:** Regardless of genetic risk, regular check-ups can lead to early detection.

## In Conclusion

The promise of genetics is profound, offering a window into our individual risks and empowering us with knowledge. However, it's essential to approach this science with a balanced perspective, understanding its potential and its limitations. With the right guidance and an integrative approach to health, we can harness the power of genetics in the broader journey of prevention.

# Genomic Testing and Personalized Prevention

Genomics, the study of all of a person's genes and their interactions, has heralded a new era in medicine. This understanding goes beyond mere genetics, which looks at individual genes, to encompass the entire genome. One of the most exciting applications of genomics is personalized prevention, particularly in the context of cancer.

# 1. What is Genomic Testing?

Genomic testing examines the entirety of an individual's DNA. This is not limited to identifying mutations in single genes but evaluates broader interactions, duplications, deletions, and other complex genetic patterns:

- **Whole-Genome Sequencing:** Examines the complete DNA sequence, providing a comprehensive genetic overview.
- **Whole-Exome Sequencing:** Focuses on the parts of the genome responsible for encoding proteins, where many disease-related mutations occur.

# 2. How Can Genomic Testing Assist in Cancer Prevention?

With the vast information gleaned from such testing, several preventive strategies can be tailored:

- **Risk Stratification:** Individuals can be classified based on their genetic risk, allowing for personalized prevention strategies.
- **Early Detection:** For those at high risk, more frequent and specific screenings can be recommended, increasing the chances of catching cancers early when they are most treatable.
- **Targeted Therapies:** If there's a known genetic risk, certain medications or treatments can be used prophylactically or in the earliest stages of cancer development.

# 3. The Advent of Personalized Medicine

The broader implications of genomic testing introduce a paradigm shift towards personalized medicine:

- **Tailored Treatment Plans:** Beyond prevention, if cancer does develop, the treatment can be customized based on an individual's genomic profile.
- **Reduced Side Effects:** By targeting treatments more precisely, patients might experience fewer adverse effects.
- **Improved Outcomes:** With more specific treatments, the chances of success can significantly increase.

# 4. Considerations in Genomic Testing

While the potential of genomic testing is vast, there are several factors to weigh:

- **Cost:** Comprehensive genomic tests can be expensive, and not all insurance plans cover them.
- **Data Overload:** The vast amount of data generated can sometimes be challenging to interpret and can lead to information that has uncertain implications.
- **Privacy Concerns:** Managing and protecting genetic data is crucial to ensure individuals' privacy is not compromised.

# 5. Ethical Implications

The power of genomic information brings forth ethical dilemmas:

- **Disclosure:** Should all information from a genomic test be shared with an individual, even if its implications aren't fully understood?
- **Consent:** Especially when testing children, is it ethical to obtain genomic information that might have implications later in life?
- **Discrimination:** There's a need to protect individuals from genetic discrimination, particularly concerning employment or insurance.

# 6. The Role of Genetic Counselors in Genomic Testing

As the complexities of genomic data increase, so does the importance of genetic counselors:

- **Interpretation:** Counselors can help distill the vast amount of information into actionable insights.
- **Guidance:** Based on an individual's genomic profile, counselors can recommend specific prevention or treatment strategies.
- **Emotional Support:** Receiving detailed genetic information can be overwhelming; counselors provide the necessary psychological support.

## In Conclusion

The field of genomics offers a transformative approach to understanding, preventing, and treating cancer. As we continue to unravel the intricacies of our genome, the prospects for personalized prevention and treatment grow. However, with these advancements come challenges and responsibilities. A thoughtful and informed approach, with the assistance of trained professionals, can ensure that we harness the power of genomics to its fullest potential, always prioritizing the well-being and autonomy of individuals.

# Ethical and Practical Considerations

The revelations that arise from genetics and genomics have undeniably propelled the medical field forward, offering a tailored approach to disease prevention and treatment. However, this powerful knowledge also introduces multifaceted ethical and practical challenges. Addressing these issues is pivotal in ensuring the responsible application of genetic information in healthcare.

## 1. Privacy and Confidentiality

With the rise of genetic testing, safeguarding an individual's genetic data becomes paramount:

- **Sensitive Information:** A person's genetic data can reveal not just about them, but potentially about their relatives as well.

- **Potential Misuse:** There's a risk that third parties (like employers or insurers) might misuse genetic information, leading to discrimination.

- **Secure Storage:** Ensuring secure and private storage of genetic data is crucial.

## 2. Informed Consent

The process of obtaining consent for genetic testing needs to be comprehensive:

- **Understanding Implications:** Individuals must be made aware of what the tests can reveal, including unexpected findings.

- **Deciding on Disclosure:** Individuals should have the autonomy to decide which results they want to be informed about.
- **Consent for Minors:** The decision to test children or adolescents, who may not fully grasp the implications, is a nuanced ethical challenge.

## 3. Return of Results

Determining which results to return to the individual presents ethical dilemmas:

- **Actionable vs. Non-actionable Results:** Should individuals receive information only on conditions that can be treated or prevented, or should they also get data about conditions with no current interventions?
- **Incidental Findings:** These are unexpected results unrelated to the initial reason for testing. Deciding on their disclosure is complex.

## 4. Genetic Testing and Family Dynamics

Genetic information doesn't just affect the individual tested:

- **Implications for Relatives:** A genetic mutation identified in one person might have implications for their family members, who may be at risk too.
- **Communication Challenges:** Deciding if, how, and when to share genetic risk information with family can be emotionally charged.
- **Family Planning:** Genetic findings can influence decisions about having children and the potential risk to offspring.

## 5. Genetic Discrimination

The potential misuse of genetic information is a significant concern:

- **Insurance Implications:** There's a fear that insurance companies might increase premiums or deny coverage based on genetic predisposition to certain diseases.

- **Employment Concerns:** Employers might discriminate based on an individual's genetic risk of developing a condition in the future.
- **Legal Protections:** While some laws prohibit genetic discrimination, they're not universal and might have loopholes.

## 6. Commercial Genetic Testing

Direct-to-consumer genetic tests have surged in popularity:

- **Accuracy and Reliability:** Not all commercial tests are held to the same standards as clinical tests, leading to potential inaccuracies.
- **Interpreting Results:** Without proper counseling, consumers might misinterpret or misjudge the implications of their results.
- **Data Sharing Concerns:** Some companies may share or sell genetic data, raising privacy issues.

## 7. Cultural and Societal Implications

Different societies and cultures view genetic information and interventions variably:

- **Cultural Sensitivity:** Respecting cultural beliefs and values concerning genetic information is essential.
- **Stigmatization:** In some cultures, known genetic mutations might lead to social stigmatization or reduced marriage prospects.

## In Conclusion

While genetics offers a wealth of information and the potential for groundbreaking preventive and therapeutic strategies, it comes with its set of ethical and practical challenges. Striking a balance between harnessing its power and respecting individual rights and societal implications is crucial. As the science progresses, ongoing dialogue, informed policies, and patient-centered care will ensure that genetics serves as a force for good in the realm of healthcare.

# Chapter 11: Alternative and Complementary Therapies

## Holistic Approaches to Prevention

As the medical landscape expands, there's an increasing recognition of the significance of holistic approaches in disease prevention, including cancer. Holistic medicine views the body, mind, and spirit as interconnected, and seeks to address all these aspects to promote overall health and well-being. In the realm of cancer prevention, various alternative and complementary therapies are being explored and integrated into traditional care.

## 1. Mind-Body Practices

These techniques emphasize the connection between the mind and body, advocating that a balanced mental state can positively influence physical health:

- **Meditation:** Regular meditation is believed to reduce stress, a known factor in numerous diseases, including cancer.
- **Yoga:** Beyond its physical benefits, yoga's emphasis on breathing and mindfulness can enhance overall well-being.
- **Tai Chi:** This ancient Chinese practice combines slow movements with breathing exercises, promoting physical and mental harmony.

## 2. Dietary and Herbal Approaches

Certain foods and herbs have been highlighted for their potential cancer-preventing properties:

- **Green Tea:** Rich in antioxidants, regular consumption is linked to a reduced risk of several cancers.
- **Turmeric:** Curcumin, the active ingredient, has been studied for its anti-inflammatory and anti-cancer properties.
- **Adaptogenic Herbs:** Herbs like Ashwagandha and Reishi are believed to boost the immune system and help the body combat stress.

## 3. Energy Therapies

The premise of energy therapies is that disruptions in the body's energy fields can lead to disease:

- **Reiki:** Practitioners believe they can channel healing energy into a patient to restore balance and health.
- **Acupuncture:** By inserting needles into specific points, it's thought to realign the body's energy and promote healing. It's also used for pain management and to alleviate treatment side effects.

## 4. Body-Based Practices

These approaches involve manipulation or movement of the body:

- **Massage Therapy:** Beyond relaxation, massage can help with lymphatic drainage, potentially aiding in toxin elimination.
- **Chiropractic Care:** By ensuring spinal alignment, chiropractors believe they can promote overall health and well-being.

## 5. Aromatherapy

Utilizing essential oils, aromatherapy believes that certain scents can influence health:

- **Lavender:** Known for its relaxation properties, it might help in reducing stress.
- **Frankincense:** Historically, it's been used for its potential healing properties.

## 6. Spiritual and Emotional Healing

Addressing emotional and spiritual well-being is foundational in holistic approaches:

- **Counseling and Psychotherapy:** Addressing emotional traumas and stressors can potentially reduce disease risk.
- **Spiritual Practices:** Whether it's prayer, attending religious services, or other spiritual practices, many believe they play a role in overall health.

## 7. Considerations in Holistic Approaches

While holistic therapies offer potential benefits, it's crucial to approach them thoughtfully:

- **Evidence Base:** Not all holistic approaches have robust scientific evidence supporting their effectiveness.
- **Integration with Traditional Care:** Always inform healthcare providers of any alternative therapies being pursued.
- **Potential Interactions:** Some herbs or supplements might interact with traditional medications or treatments.

## In Conclusion

Holistic approaches to cancer prevention emphasize the interconnectedness of the body, mind, and spirit. By addressing all these facets, the belief is that one can create an optimal environment for health and well-being, potentially reducing the risk of diseases, including cancer. As research continues, the integration of these therapies with traditional medicine can offer a comprehensive strategy, ensuring that patients receive the best of both worlds in their quest for health.

# Herbal Supplements and Cancer Prevention

The allure of nature's remedies has persisted throughout human history. In recent decades, there has been a resurgence of interest in herbal supplements, particularly for their potential role in preventing or even treating various ailments, including cancer. While many of these herbs have traditional backings and some preliminary scientific evidence, it's crucial to approach their use with informed caution.

# 1. Turmeric (Curcumin)

**Background:** Turmeric, a golden-hued spice, is a staple in Asian cuisine and Ayurvedic medicine. Curcumin is its active ingredient.

**Potential Benefits:** Curcumin has exhibited anti-inflammatory, antioxidant, and even direct anti-cancer effects in some laboratory studies. Its potential roles in preventing tumor growth, invasion, and angiogenesis have been explored.

**Considerations:** While promising, it's essential to note that curcumin's bioavailability is low, meaning it's not easily absorbed in the digestive tract. Some supplements include piperine to enhance absorption.

# 2. Green Tea (EGCG)

**Background:** Green tea, derived from the *Camellia sinensis* plant, is rich in polyphenols, particularly epigallocatechin gallate (EGCG).

**Potential Benefits:** EGCG has shown anti-cancer properties in multiple studies, potentially preventing cancer cell growth and inducing apoptosis (programmed cell death).

**Considerations:** Excessive green tea or concentrated supplements can impact liver function, so moderation and monitoring are crucial.

# 3. Milk Thistle (Silymarin)

**Background:** Used traditionally for liver disorders, milk thistle contains the active compound silymarin.

**Potential Benefits:** Some studies suggest that silymarin can inhibit cancer cell growth and multiplication, especially in breast, cervical, and prostate cancers.

**Considerations:** Milk thistle might interact with some medications, so consulting with a healthcare professional before use is advisable.

## 4. Astragalus

**Background:** A staple in traditional Chinese medicine, astragalus is believed to stimulate the immune system.

**Potential Benefits:** Some evidence suggests it can boost the effects of certain chemotherapy drugs and reduce their side effects. It might also inhibit tumor growth.

**Considerations:** Astragalus can interact with medications, especially those affecting the immune system, so ensure to discuss its use with a doctor.

## 5. Graviola (Soursop)

**Background:** Graviola has traditionally been used for a range of health conditions.

**Potential Benefits:** Some laboratory studies suggest that graviola extracts can slow the growth of cancer cells, but human studies are lacking.

**Considerations:** There are concerns about neurotoxicity with prolonged use, and it can interfere with blood pressure medications.

## 6. Echinacea

**Background:** Commonly used to prevent colds, echinacea is also explored for its potential anti-cancer properties.

**Potential Benefits:** Some compounds in echinacea might stimulate the immune system and potentially slow tumor growth.

**Considerations:** Allergic reactions can occur, and those with autoimmune diseases should be cautious.

## In Conclusion

Herbal supplements offer a glimmer of hope in the vast arena of cancer prevention. However, several critical considerations come into play:

- **Research Gaps:** While some laboratory studies are promising, human trials are often limited or lacking. It's crucial to differentiate between lab results and real-world effectiveness.
- **Interactions:** Herbs can interact with traditional medications, potentially reducing their efficacy or causing side effects.
- **Quality:** The quality and concentration of herbal supplements can vary widely between brands.

It's essential to remember that no single herb or supplement can "cure" or "prevent" cancer independently. However, they might play a role within a broader preventive strategy. Always consult with healthcare professionals before incorporating new supplements into a regimen.

# Mind-Body Practices

In the vast realm of holistic medicine, mind-body practices have garnered significant attention for their potential role in preventing and managing diseases, including cancer. These practices, rooted in ancient traditions, emphasize the profound interconnection between our mental and physical states. Let's explore some popular mind-body practices and understand their potential benefits and considerations.

## 1. Meditation

**Background:** Meditation is a practice that encourages mental clarity, calmness, and emotional positivity. Various types include mindfulness meditation, transcendental meditation, and loving-kindness meditation.

**Potential Benefits:** Regular meditation can reduce stress hormones, lower blood pressure, and enhance immune function. It's also linked to positive changes in the brain, such as increased gray matter density in areas related to memory and emotional processing.

**Considerations:** Meditation requires practice and patience. Finding a quiet space and dedicating a set time each day can help establish a routine.

## 2. Yoga

**Background:** Originating in ancient India, yoga combines physical postures, breathing exercises, and meditation to promote holistic well-being.

**Potential Benefits:** Yoga can enhance flexibility, balance, and strength. Moreover, its stress-reducing effects have been linked to decreased inflammation and improved immune function. It can also improve sleep quality, a vital factor in overall health and cancer prevention.

**Considerations:** Not all yoga styles are suitable for everyone. Individuals should choose a style that matches their fitness level and always consult with a healthcare professional if they have pre-existing health conditions.

## 3. Tai Chi

**Background:** A graceful form of exercise developed in ancient China, Tai Chi involves slow, flowing movements paired with deep breathing.

**Potential Benefits:** Tai Chi can boost balance and muscular strength. Its meditative nature can reduce stress, lower blood pressure, and improve sleep. Studies have also hinted at its potential to boost the immune system and decrease inflammation.

**Considerations:** It's advisable to learn Tai Chi from qualified instructors to ensure proper technique and gain maximum benefits.

## 4. Guided Imagery

**Background:** This technique involves visualizing positive images, scenes, or experiences to induce physical relaxation and emotional calmness.

**Potential Benefits:** Guided imagery can reduce stress, alleviate pain, improve mood, and even bolster the immune response. It's particularly beneficial for patients undergoing cancer treatments, helping them manage treatment-related anxiety and side effects.

**Considerations:** While generally safe, individuals with a history of trauma should approach guided imagery with caution, as it can sometimes trigger distressing memories.

## 5. Biofeedback

**Background:** Biofeedback trains individuals to control physiological processes such as heart rate, muscle tension, and blood pressure. Using electronic monitoring, users receive real-time data on these bodily functions.

**Potential Benefits:** Biofeedback can enhance relaxation, reduce pain, and manage stress-related disorders. By understanding their body's involuntary responses, individuals can learn to make voluntary changes for better health.

**Considerations:** This practice requires specialized equipment and training, usually under the guidance of trained therapists.

## In Conclusion

Mind-body practices embrace the philosophy that our mental state profoundly influences our physical health. While research continues to explore the full range of benefits, preliminary evidence strongly supports their integration into a comprehensive health regimen.

Incorporating these practices doesn't mean abandoning conventional medical treatments, especially when addressing severe diseases like cancer. Instead, they can complement traditional approaches, providing a holistic strategy that addresses both the body and mind. Before starting any new practice, consulting with a healthcare professional ensures it's suitable and safe.

# Chapter 12: Navigating the Healthcare System

## Building a Relationship with Healthcare Providers

Establishing a trusting and collaborative relationship with healthcare providers is fundamental for anyone invested in their long-term health, especially when considering cancer prevention and treatment. A strong patient-provider partnership can greatly influence outcomes, enhance understanding, and foster a sense of security. Here's a guide to building and maintaining that pivotal relationship.

### 1. Open Communication

**Background:** An open line of communication is the backbone of any relationship, particularly one as crucial as that between patient and provider.

**Importance:** Freely sharing symptoms, concerns, and lifestyle habits ensures that the provider has a comprehensive view of the patient's health. It also ensures that patients fully understand medical advice, diagnoses, and treatment options.

**Tips:** Always come prepared with questions for appointments. Consider keeping a health journal to track symptoms or concerns.

### 2. Mutual Respect

**Background:** Respect is a two-way street. While patients should expect respect from their healthcare provider, they should also give it in return.

**Importance:** Mutual respect fosters a safe environment where both parties feel valued, heard, and understood. This dynamic encourages openness and trust.

**Tips:** Understand that providers may have constraints (like time limits per appointment). Be punctual for appointments, and if you have a lot to discuss, consider notifying the clinic in advance.

## 3. Active Participation

**Background:** Being an active participant means taking an interest in one's health and being proactive about it.

**Importance:** Active involvement empowers patients to make informed decisions, adhere to medical advice, and play a role in shaping their health journey.

**Tips:** Research (from reputable sources) about any diagnoses or treatments. Ask for clarifications whenever something is unclear.

## 4. Continuity of Care

**Background:** Continuity of care refers to consistent care provided over time, typically by the same healthcare professional or team.

**Importance:** It ensures that the provider is familiar with the patient's medical history, leading to more personalized care. It also reduces redundancy in tests and miscommunications.

**Tips:** Try to schedule regular check-ups with the same provider or clinic. If you must see a specialist, ensure they communicate with your primary care provider.

## 5. Honesty and Transparency

**Background:** Honesty goes beyond sharing symptoms; it includes being transparent about lifestyle choices, adherence to medications, and more.

**Importance:** Being truthful ensures that healthcare providers have an accurate picture, leading to more appropriate care. It also avoids potential complications.

**Tips:** If there are barriers to following medical advice (e.g., medication costs), discuss them openly with the provider. They might offer solutions or alternatives.

## 6. Feedback and Advocacy

**Background:** Like any professional, healthcare providers can benefit from feedback. Patients also have the right to advocate for their health.

**Importance:** Feedback helps providers improve their service. Advocacy ensures that patients receive the care they need and deserve.

**Tips:** If you feel a diagnosis or treatment isn't fitting, seek a second opinion. Constructive feedback, both positive and negative, can usually be provided through clinic surveys or direct communication.

## In Conclusion

Building a relationship with healthcare providers is akin to cultivating a partnership. It requires effort, understanding, and patience from both parties. In the complex maze of the healthcare system, particularly in areas as intricate as cancer prevention and treatment, this bond can serve as a guiding light, illuminating the path towards better health outcomes, mutual trust, and peace of mind.

# Advocating for One's Health

Advocacy, at its heart, is about taking action on behalf of a cause or a particular group. When it comes to healthcare, advocating for oneself is about understanding one's rights as a patient, seeking out the best care possible, and taking proactive steps to ensure one's voice is heard. As patients navigate the healthcare system, particularly in the realm of cancer prevention and care, this self-advocacy becomes an invaluable skill. Let's delve into how one can champion their health effectively.

## 1. Educate Yourself

**Background:** Knowledge is power. By understanding your health condition, available treatments, and preventative measures, you become an informed advocate.

**Importance:** When you're well-informed, you can communicate more effectively with healthcare providers, ask relevant questions, and make decisions that align with your values and priorities.

**Tips:** Seek information from credible sources, such as renowned health organizations or peer-reviewed studies. Don't hesitate to ask your doctor for resources or reading recommendations.

## 2. Know Your Rights

**Background:** Every patient has rights, which may include the right to informed consent, privacy, and receiving a second opinion.

**Importance:** Being aware of your rights ensures that you receive respectful and appropriate care. It also means you're better equipped to address any issues or concerns that arise.

**Tips:** Familiarize yourself with patient rights specific to your country or region. Many hospitals and clinics have this information readily available.

## 3. Keep Detailed Health Records

**Background:** Maintaining a comprehensive record of your medical history, treatments, medications, and test results is essential.

**Importance:** Accurate health records can prevent redundant tests, help new or specialist doctors understand your health background quickly, and enable you to monitor and understand changes in your health.

**Tips:** Organize records chronologically. Consider digital tools or apps designed for this purpose. Always request copies of test results.

## 4. Develop Strong Communication Skills

**Background:** Effective communication is the cornerstone of self-advocacy.

**Importance:** By expressing concerns, asking questions, and clarifying doubts in a clear manner, patients can foster a collaborative relationship with healthcare providers, ensuring they're partners in the care journey.

**Tips:** Prepare questions before appointments. Practice active listening. Don't hesitate to ask for clarifications if something is unclear.

## 5. Seek a Second Opinion

**Background:** If ever in doubt about a diagnosis, treatment plan, or any aspect of care, it's within a patient's rights to seek another professional opinion.

**Importance:** Second opinions can offer reassurance, provide alternative treatment options, or shed new light on a health issue.

**Tips:** Choose a doctor who specializes in the relevant field and ensure they have access to your medical records for a comprehensive review.

## 6. Find a Support System

**Background:** Advocacy can sometimes feel overwhelming. Having a support system, whether it's family, friends, or patient support groups, can make the journey smoother.

**Importance:** Support systems offer emotional backing, help process information, and sometimes even accompany patients to appointments, providing an additional set of ears and eyes.

**Tips:** Explore local or online support groups. Consider designating a trusted individual to be your health advocate, especially during critical care phases.

## In Conclusion

Advocating for one's health is not about confrontation but about collaboration. It's about ensuring the patient's voice is central in healthcare decisions. Especially in complex areas like cancer care, where decisions can influence quality of life and treatment outcomes, self-advocacy becomes both a responsibility and a right. As patients become active participants in their care journey, the path to optimal health becomes clearer and more navigable.

# Health Insurance and Coverage Considerations

Navigating the intricacies of health insurance can be daunting. Yet, understanding insurance and its implications on medical care is vital, especially when considering preventive measures and treatments for conditions like cancer. While health insurance structures and specifics vary by country and provider, some general principles can guide individuals in making informed decisions. Here's a deeper dive into health insurance considerations for optimal health management.

## 1. Understanding Your Policy

**Background:** Every health insurance policy provides a defined set of benefits. These typically encompass doctor visits, hospital stays, preventive care, prescription drugs, and other essentials.

**Importance:** Knowing the specifics of your policy helps in anticipating out-of-pocket costs and ensuring necessary treatments are covered.

**Tips:** Always read the 'Summary of Benefits and Coverage' of your plan. If unclear about certain terms, consult with the insurance provider or an insurance broker.

## 2. Preventive Services Coverage

**Background:** Many insurance plans, especially after global drives towards preventive healthcare, cover routine screenings and check-ups.

**Importance:** Regular screenings can detect potential health issues, like cancer, early, making treatment more effective. Ensuring these are covered minimizes financial strain.

**Tips:** Review your policy to understand which screenings are covered and how often. Remember, early detection can save lives and reduce treatment costs.

## 3. Specialist Visits and Referrals

**Background:** Some insurance plans require a referral from a primary care physician (PCP) before seeing a specialist.

**Importance:** Knowing the referral process prevents unexpected costs and ensures seamless care, especially when dealing with diseases that require specialist input.

**Tips:** Establish a relationship with a PCP who understands your health history and can guide you to the right specialists when needed.

## 4. Prescription Drug Coverage

**Background:** Medications, including cancer drugs, can be costly. Insurance policies have 'formularies' or lists of covered drugs.

**Importance:** Understanding drug coverage can influence treatment decisions and help manage expenses.

**Tips:** If a required medication isn't covered, discuss alternative options with your healthcare provider or explore patient assistance programs.

## 5. Out-of-Network Care

**Background:** Health insurance plans have networks of preferred providers. Receiving care outside this network can be more expensive.

**Importance:** In emergencies or for specialized care, patients may need out-of-network services. Knowing the costs involved can prevent financial surprises.

**Tips:** If seeking a second opinion or specialized care, check if the provider is in-network. In unavoidable out-of-network situations, negotiate costs beforehand.

## 6. Annual Maximums and Deductibles

**Background:** Many insurance policies have deductibles (amounts you pay before insurance kicks in) and annual out-of-pocket maximums.

**Importance:** Budgeting for potential health costs becomes easier when you know these figures.

**Tips:** Set aside funds to cover deductibles. Once you hit your annual maximum, the insurance typically covers 100% of allowed amounts for covered services.

## 7. International and Travel Coverage

**Background:** If traveling or residing temporarily in another country, your regular insurance might not cover healthcare costs.

**Importance:** Medical emergencies or the need for routine care can arise anytime. Being prepared prevents significant financial distress.

**Tips:** Consider purchasing travel or international health insurance. Always carry a copy of your insurance details when traveling.

## In Conclusion

While health insurance complexities can seem overwhelming, a proactive approach to understanding coverage can make all the difference. As the old adage goes, "knowledge is power." Being informed empowers individuals to make the best decisions for their health while managing costs. Especially in the realm of cancer prevention and care, where timely interventions matter immensely, having the backing of a robust insurance plan can be both a comfort and a necessity.

# Chapter 13: Cancer Myths and Misconceptions

## Debunking Common Myths

As with many health-related topics, there are numerous myths and misconceptions surrounding cancer. While some of these myths are benign, others can lead to unnecessary fear, stigma, or even misguided decisions regarding prevention and treatment. Let's debunk some of the most pervasive cancer myths:

### 1. Myth: Cancer is Always Fatal

**Truth:** Many cancers are highly treatable, especially when detected early. The survival rate for many types of cancer has increased over the years due to advancements in diagnosis and treatment methods.

### 2. Myth: Cancer is Contagious

**Truth:** With very few exceptions (like transplant patients receiving an organ from a cancer-afflicted donor), cancer is not contagious. You can't "catch" cancer from someone else.

### 3. Myth: Cell Phones Cause Cancer

**Truth:** Current research suggests that cell phones do not emit enough radiation to cause DNA damage that can lead to cancer. While it's good to be cautious, using cell phones does not seem to increase cancer risk.

### 4. Myth: Cancer Surgery Causes Cancer to Spread

**Truth:** Surgery, when done by experienced surgeons following standard protocols, does not cause cancer to spread. In fact, surgery is often a primary method to remove tumors and stop cancer growth.

## 5. Myth: Artificial Sweeteners Cause Cancer

**Truth:** Numerous studies have been conducted on artificial sweeteners like aspartame, saccharin, and sucralose. To date, there's no conclusive scientific evidence linking these sweeteners to cancer when consumed in regular dietary amounts.

## 6. Myth: Only Smokers Get Lung Cancer

**Truth:** While smoking significantly increases the risk of lung cancer, non-smokers can also develop the disease. Other risk factors include exposure to radon gas, secondhand smoke, certain chemicals, and family history.

## 7. Myth: Deodorants and Antiperspirants Cause Breast Cancer

**Truth:** There is no solid evidence linking the use of underarm deodorants or antiperspirants to breast cancer. This myth likely originated due to some products containing parabens, but most major studies have found no direct link between these products and breast cancer.

## 8. Myth: Biopsies Can Spread Cancer

**Truth:** When done properly, a biopsy – which involves taking a small tissue sample for testing – does not cause cancer to spread. Biopsies are crucial for diagnosing cancer and determining its type and stage.

## 9. Myth: Cancer Has a Singular Cure

**Truth:** Cancer is not a single disease but a collection of related diseases. Consequently, it's unlikely there will ever be a "one-size-fits-all" cure. Treatments are tailored to the type, stage, and location of the cancer, as well as the patient's health and preferences.

## 10. Myth: Sharks Don't Get Cancer

**Truth:** This myth has been used to promote shark cartilage as a cancer treatment. In reality, sharks can and do get cancer. Moreover, no scientific evidence supports the efficacy of shark cartilage as a cancer treatment.

## In Conclusion

Misinformation can be harmful. When it comes to health and particularly something as significant as cancer, it's crucial to base our knowledge and decisions on science-backed information. Myths can create unnecessary fear or provide false hope. By seeking reliable sources, consulting with healthcare professionals, and staying informed, individuals can better navigate the complexities of cancer and its prevention.

# How to Stay Informed

In today's information age, we are inundated with a constant stream of news, articles, videos, and social media posts. While access to information has never been more abundant, this also brings the challenge of discerning reliable sources from misleading or outright false ones. When it comes to health and cancer-related matters, the stakes are high. Misinformation can lead to poor health choices, misplaced fears, or misguided treatments. Here's how you can stay informed and ensure that the information you rely on is accurate and trustworthy:

## 1. Rely on Established Health Organizations

**Trusted Sources:** Organizations such as the World Health Organization (WHO), Centers for Disease Control and Prevention (CDC), American Cancer Society (ACS), and National Cancer Institute (NCI) offer a wealth of up-to-date and peer-reviewed information on various health topics, including cancer.

## 2. Be Skeptical of Sensational Headlines

**Critical Reading:** News outlets sometimes use sensational or exaggerated headlines to attract readers. It's essential to read the full article, not just the headline, and determine if the content supports the claims made in the title.

## 3. Understand the Nature of Scientific Studies

**Interpreting Research:** Not all studies are created equal. Understand the difference between observational studies, clinical trials, case studies, and more. Recognize that early-stage research, especially studies done on animals, may not directly translate to human application.

## 4. Check for Peer-Reviewed Sources

**Reliability Matters:** Peer-reviewed journals require that experts in the field evaluate articles before publication. This process ensures the research is of high quality and free from major errors. If an article or study hasn't been peer-reviewed, it's wise to approach it with caution.

## 5. Be Cautious with Anecdotal Evidence

**Personal Stories vs. Scientific Evidence:** While personal stories can be compelling, they are not a substitute for comprehensive scientific research. Anecdotes can provide insight but should not form the sole basis for health decisions.

## 6. Diversify Your Information Sources

**Broaden Your Horizons:** Relying on a single source or type of media can give a skewed perspective. By diversifying where and how you get your information, you'll have a more rounded and balanced view of the topic at hand.

## 7. Engage with Healthcare Professionals

**Expert Insight:** Doctors, nurses, and other healthcare professionals have trained extensively in their fields. They can provide context, clear up misunderstandings, and guide you towards reliable resources. Don't hesitate to ask them questions or seek their opinion on something you've read or heard.

## 8. Be Wary of Conflicts of Interest

**Hidden Agendas:** Sometimes, articles or studies may have underlying motives, such as promoting a product or service. Check the funding source of research studies and be alert to potential biases.

## 9. Participate in Workshops and Seminars

**Continued Learning:** Many hospitals, clinics, universities, and community centers offer workshops and seminars on health topics, including cancer. These events can be an excellent opportunity to learn directly from experts and ask questions.

## 10. Stay Updated

**Ongoing Research:** The field of medicine, and particularly cancer research, is continually evolving. What was considered best practice a few years ago might have been updated or refined. Regularly revisit trusted sources to stay on top of the latest findings and recommendations.

## In Conclusion

Staying informed is an active process that requires discernment and a willingness to seek out the best and most accurate information. With the plethora of sources available, armed with critical thinking and a proactive approach, you can navigate the vast seas of information and stay well-informed about cancer and its prevention.

# Evaluating Sources of Information

The quest for knowledge about cancer can lead us through a maze of information sources. From personal blogs to scientific journals, the spectrum of available materials is vast and varied. However, it's crucial to remember that not all sources are created equal. Some might offer objective, evidence-based findings, while others might be biased or based on unsubstantiated claims. Here's a guide to help you critically evaluate sources of information:

## 1. Authorship: Who Wrote It?

**Credentials Matter:** Look for the author's qualifications. A piece written by a doctor or scientist in the field of oncology, for instance, will likely be more reliable than an anonymous internet post. Reputable publications typically provide a brief bio of the author, highlighting their expertise.

## 2. Source: Where Was It Published?

**Reputable Platforms:** Articles or studies published in peer-reviewed journals, established health organizations' websites (like the WHO or CDC), and academic institutions are generally trustworthy. Be wary of personal blogs, unverified news websites, or sources that lack transparency about their origins.

## 3. Citations: Are Claims Supported?

**Backing Evidence:** Reliable articles provide references to the studies or sources they cite. This allows readers to verify the claims and delve deeper if they wish. A piece that makes sweeping statements without any supporting evidence should raise red flags.

## 4. Date of Publication: Is It Current?

**Timeliness Counts:** Especially in fields like medicine, where new research is continuously emerging, it's essential to ensure the information is up-to-date. While an older source might still contain valuable insights, always cross-check to see if there have been any recent developments or updates on the subject.

## 5. Bias and Objectivity: Is There an Underlying Agenda?

**Detecting Bias:** Does the article seem to push a particular product, service, or viewpoint aggressively? If a piece feels more like an advertisement than an informative article, be cautious. Additionally, check if the source has any affiliations that might influence its content.

## 6. Language and Tone: Is It Sensational or Objective?

**Stay Grounded:** Be skeptical of articles that use sensationalistic language, make grandiose promises, or rely heavily on emotional anecdotes rather than factual evidence. A balanced, objective tone is a hallmark of credible reporting.

## 7. Peer Review: Has It Been Evaluated by Experts?

**Quality Control:** Peer-reviewed journals are considered the gold standard in academic publishing. Before an article appears in such a journal, it undergoes a rigorous review by experts in the field. This process ensures the research's validity and reliability.

## 8. Public Consensus vs. Expert Consensus

**Popularity Doesn't Equal Accuracy:** Just because a particular viewpoint is widespread doesn't mean it's accurate. Sometimes, myths or misconceptions can become popularly accepted truths. Always prioritize expert consensus over public opinion.

## 9. Cross-reference with Multiple Sources

**Diversify Your Reading:** Don't rely on a single source for your information. If you come across a claim or piece of data, check it against other reputable sources. This cross-referencing can help confirm the information's accuracy and give you a more comprehensive understanding.

## 10. Trust Your Instincts

**Intuition Matters:** If something doesn't feel right or seems too good to be true, it's worth taking a moment to dig deeper. Your intuition, combined with critical thinking skills, can be a powerful tool in evaluating information.

## In Conclusion

In our modern age, where information is at our fingertips, the ability to critically evaluate sources is more important than ever. By developing a discerning eye and being proactive about where and how you gather information, you can ensure that your knowledge about cancer and its prevention is both comprehensive and accurate.

# Chapter 14: Conclusion: Embracing a Proactive Lifestyle

## Key Takeaways

As we reach the conclusion of our journey through understanding cancer prevention and its relationship with aging, let's reflect upon the essential learnings that we've acquired. Embracing a proactive lifestyle not only diminishes the risk of developing cancer but also contributes to a richer, healthier life. Here are the salient points to remember:

## 1. The Interconnection of Aging and Cancer

**Understanding the Link:** As we age, the risk of developing cancer increases, primarily due to accumulated genetic mutations, weakened immune systems, and lifestyle choices made over the years. Recognizing this correlation equips us to be more vigilant and proactive in our health endeavors.

## 2. Lifelong Prevention

**Every Stage Matters:** Cancer prevention is not a one-time task; it's a lifelong commitment. From childhood to our senior years, every life stage offers unique challenges and opportunities for cancer prevention.

## 3. Nutrition is Paramount

**Eat to Beat Cancer:** Our dietary choices significantly influence our cancer risk. Prioritizing whole foods, vegetables, fruits, and reducing processed or red meat intake can make a considerable difference. Additionally, understanding the importance of antioxidants, phytochemicals, and proper hydration underscores the role nutrition plays in overall health.

## 4. Move Your Body

**The Power of Physical Activity:** Regular exercise does more than just keep you fit; it actively reduces the risk of various cancers. As we age, ensuring that our physical activity aligns with our capabilities while prioritizing safety becomes even more crucial.

## 5. The Environment's Silent Role

**Guard Against Hidden Dangers:** From UV exposure to household chemicals, our environment is rife with potential carcinogens. Being aware and making informed choices can significantly reduce our risk.

## 6. Screenings: The Power of Early Detection

**Timely Interventions:** Regular health screenings and check-ups can catch abnormalities early, making treatment more effective and often less invasive. Understanding which screenings are essential at different life stages ensures that we remain one step ahead.

## 7. Mental and Emotional Wellbeing

**Health Beyond the Physical:** Stress, lack of sleep, and poor mental health can indirectly contribute to cancer development by weakening our immune system and prompting poor lifestyle choices. Prioritizing mental and emotional health is as crucial as physical wellbeing.

## 8. Genetic Insights

**Personalized Prevention:** Understanding our genetic predispositions can offer tailored prevention strategies. While genetics is not destiny, being aware of potential risks can guide more informed health decisions.

## 9. Complementary Therapies

**Beyond Conventional Medicine:** While traditional medicine offers a robust framework for prevention and treatment, complementary therapies can provide additional tools for those seeking holistic approaches.

## 10. Navigating Healthcare

**Be Your Best Advocate:** Building strong relationships with healthcare providers, understanding health insurance nuances, and advocating for one's health rights are foundational to navigating the healthcare system effectively.

## 11. Staying Informed and Critical

**Knowledge is Power:** In an age of information overload, discerning between myths and facts about cancer is crucial. Equip yourself with the skills to evaluate sources and stay updated with the latest in cancer research.

## 12. Proactivity is Key

**Take Charge of Your Health:** Prevention is always better than cure. A proactive approach, encompassing regular check-ups, a balanced diet, consistent exercise, and mental wellness practices, lays the foundation for a healthier future.

## In Closing

Your health journey is uniquely yours, and while genetics and environment play roles, your choices have significant power. As you move forward, armed with the knowledge from this book, remember that every day presents an opportunity to make choices that align with a healthier, more vibrant life. Embrace the journey, celebrate the small victories, and remember: prevention is an act of self-love.

# Personal Action Plan

As we conclude our exploration into cancer prevention and the intricacies of aging, it's vital to translate the knowledge gained into actionable steps. A personal action plan serves as a tangible roadmap, guiding you in integrating these preventive measures into your daily life. Here's a guide to help you create and implement your action plan:

# 1. Self-Assessment

**Reflect on Your Lifestyle:** Begin by taking a moment to assess your current lifestyle. Consider your diet, physical activity, stress levels, and any exposures to potential carcinogens. Recognizing areas for improvement is the first step.

# 2. Dietary Changes

**Prioritize Whole Foods:** Commit to incorporating more fruits, vegetables, whole grains, and lean proteins into your meals.

**Limit Processed Foods:** Gradually reduce your intake of processed meats, sugary beverages, and overly processed snacks.

**Stay Hydrated:** Ensure you're drinking ample water daily, adjusting for physical activity and environmental factors.

# 3. Physical Activity

**Set Clear Goals:** Whether it's walking 10,000 steps a day, attending a weekly yoga class, or hitting the gym three times a week, define your fitness objectives.

**Consistency Over Intensity:** It's more important to be consistent in your physical activity than to have sporadic intense workouts. Find a routine you enjoy and can maintain.

# 4. Regular Check-ups and Screenings

**Schedule in Advance:** Plan your yearly check-ups and necessary screenings based on your age and risk factors. Mark them on your calendar or set reminders.

**Stay Informed:** Ensure you're aware of the screenings recommended for your age group and any personal risk factors.

# 5. Mental and Emotional Wellbeing

**Mindfulness Practices:** Incorporate practices like meditation or deep breathing exercises into your routine to manage stress.

**Seek Support:** If you find yourself struggling emotionally or mentally, consider seeking professional support or joining a support group.

## 6. Environmental Changes

**Audit Your Home:** Examine household products for potential carcinogens and consider natural alternatives.

**Practice Safe Sun:** Use sunscreens, wear protective clothing, and avoid peak UV exposure times to protect against skin cancer.

## 7. Stay Educated

**Continuous Learning:** Medicine and science are ever-evolving fields. Dedicate some time every few months to catch up on the latest research and recommendations in cancer prevention.

**Evaluate Information Sources:** Remember to approach new information critically and consider its source.

## 8. Genetics and Personal History

**Understand Your Risks:** If you have a family history of cancer or other risk factors, consider genetic counseling or testing.

**Tailor Your Plan:** Use your genetic and personal history information to modify your action plan accordingly.

## 9. Holistic and Complementary Therapies

**Research and Explore:** If you're interested in alternative therapies, do your research and consult with professionals to ensure they complement your overall prevention strategy.

## 10. Advocacy and Community

**Join a Community:** Engage with support groups or communities focused on health and cancer prevention. Sharing experiences and knowledge can be empowering.

**Advocate:** Use your voice to advocate for health policies and initiatives in your community that support cancer prevention.

## Implementing Your Plan

Creating a plan is just the first step. Implementation requires dedication, consistency, and periodic reassessments. As life changes, your action plan may need adjustments. Celebrate the milestones, no matter how small, and remember that every positive step is a move towards a healthier future.

Remember, this journey is personal. While guidance is beneficial, it's essential to listen to your body, consult with healthcare professionals, and make informed choices that align with your unique needs and circumstances.

# Hope for the Future

As we conclude our comprehensive exploration into the multifaceted world of cancer prevention and the aging process, it's essential to step back and look forward with hope. Understanding cancer, its complexities, and the ways in which we can mitigate its risk might be overwhelming, but it's a testament to the strides humanity has taken in medical science and public awareness.

## 1. Progress in Medical Science

**Advancements in Research:** Every year, countless research studies are conducted around the world, leading to breakthroughs in our understanding of cancer. These discoveries aren't just academic; they have practical applications that have, over time, improved early detection rates, treatment modalities, and post-treatment quality of life.

**Personalized Medicine:** With the emergence of genomic sequencing and personalized medicine, treatment and prevention are becoming more tailored to individual patients. This approach optimizes results and minimizes unnecessary interventions, making medical care more efficient and patient-centric.

## 2. Global Awareness and Collaboration

**Increased Global Awareness:** Cancer prevention is no longer a topic limited to medical professionals. With global campaigns, awareness days, and easily accessible information, the average individual is more informed than ever about the importance of preventive measures.

**Collaborative Efforts:** Many nations collaborate on cancer research, combining resources, expertise, and data to understand the disease better and devise novel solutions. This spirit of international cooperation is accelerating breakthroughs and their real-world applications.

## 3. Embracing Preventive Lifestyles

**Shifting Mindsets:** More people are recognizing the significance of a proactive approach to health. By adopting a lifestyle that's centered around prevention, we're not just reducing the risk of cancer but also bolstering our defenses against various other diseases and conditions.

**Accessible Resources:** From apps that track nutrition and physical activity to online platforms offering meditation and stress-relief tools, taking charge of one's health has never been easier.

## 4. Empowerment through Education

**Knowledge is Power:** With resources like this book and many others, individuals can equip themselves with knowledge, fostering an empowered approach to health decisions.

**The Role of Institutions:** Schools, universities, and other institutions are increasingly incorporating health education into their curriculums, ensuring future generations grow up with an ingrained understanding of wellness and prevention.

## 5. The Role of Technology

**Innovative Diagnostics:** Technological advancements are continually improving diagnostic techniques, allowing for earlier and more accurate cancer detection.

**Digital Support Communities:** Through the internet, individuals can find communities, support groups, and resources tailored to their specific needs and concerns. These platforms provide invaluable emotional and informational support.

## 6. Nature and Complementary Therapies

**Back to Basics:** There's a global movement towards embracing nature, organic foods, and natural living as a way to counteract the pitfalls of modern lifestyles that might increase disease risk.

**Holistic Health:** Complementary therapies, from acupuncture to herbal medicine, are being studied and integrated into conventional medical practice, offering patients a more holistic approach to health and wellness.

## Looking Ahead with Optimism

While the fight against cancer continues, there's undeniable hope on the horizon. The combination of scientific advancements, global collaboration, and individual empowerment is paving the way for a brighter, healthier future. Each one of us plays a role in this narrative of progress. By staying informed, making conscious choices, and supporting broader health initiatives, we can collectively make a difference.

Remember, every step, no matter how small, that we take towards understanding and preventing cancer, contributes to a larger global movement towards health, longevity, and wellbeing.

# Appendix A: Resources and Support Groups

Living with the knowledge of cancer risk, undergoing screenings, or navigating the complexities of a diagnosis can be an overwhelming experience. Fortunately, numerous resources and support groups are available to assist individuals at every stage of their journey, from prevention to survivorship. Here, we outline some of the most notable organizations and tools that offer invaluable assistance.

## 1. General Cancer Resources

- **American Cancer Society (ACS):** One of the most recognized organizations globally, the ACS offers a wealth of information on different cancer types, research, treatment, and more. Their website provides patient support, caregiver advice, and recovery resources.

  - Website: https://www.cancer.org

- **World Cancer Research Fund (WCRF):** An international organization that emphasizes the connection between diet, nutrition, and cancer. Their resources provide insights into cancer prevention through lifestyle changes.

  - Website: https://www.wcrf.org

## 2. Cancer Prevention and Early Detection

- **Cancer.Net:** Sponsored by the American Society of Clinical Oncology, this site offers guidance on prevention, detection, and treatment, complete with doctor-approved patient information.

  - Website: https://www.cancer.net

- **National Cancer Institute (NCI):** The NCI provides detailed information on cancer types, treatments, and research initiatives. Their focus on early detection and prevention is especially beneficial.

  - Website: https://www.cancer.gov

## 3. Support Groups and Communities

- **Cancer Support Community (CSC):** This global nonprofit network offers a comprehensive range of support services, including counseling, support groups, education, and healthy lifestyle programs.

  - Website: https://www.cancersupportcommunity.org

- **CancerCare:** Providing free professional counseling, support groups, educational workshops, publications, and financial assistance, CancerCare has been a mainstay for patients, survivors, and caregivers.

  - Website: https://www.cancercare.org

## 4. Specialized Cancer Resources

- **BreastCancer.org:** A dedicated platform for those affected by breast cancer, this site offers medical insights, personal stories, and community support.

  - Website: https://www.breastcancer.org

- **Prostate Cancer Foundation:** A leading organization for prostate cancer research and patient support, offering detailed information and resources for patients and caregivers.

  - Website: https://www.pcf.org

## 5. Resources for Caregivers

- Family Caregiver Alliance (FCA):

Recognizing the unique challenges faced by caregivers, the FCA offers resources, advice, and support tailored to those caring for someone with cancer or other chronic conditions.

- Website: https://www.caregiver.org

## 6. Survivorship and Recovery

- LIVESTRONG:

Known globally for its advocacy, LIVESTRONG provides tools, resources, and programs for cancer survivors, helping them navigate post-treatment life.

- Website: https://www.livestrong.org

## 7. Genetics and Cancer Risk

- FORCE (Facing Our Risk of Cancer Empowered):

For individuals and families affected by hereditary breast, ovarian, and related cancers, FORCE offers resources, community support, and advocacy initiatives.

- Website: https://www.facingourrisk.org

## In Conclusion

The road to understanding, preventing, and coping with cancer is not one that anyone should walk alone. With the wealth of resources and communities available, individuals can find the knowledge, support, and camaraderie they need. Remember, reaching out for assistance or just for a listening ear can make all the difference.

# Appendix B: Recommended Readings and References

A journey through understanding, preventing, and coping with cancer is deeply personal but also widely studied. For those interested in expanding their knowledge or seeking further insights, here is a curated list of recommended readings and references spanning various facets of cancer, from scientific journals to personal memoirs.

## 1. Scientific and Medical References

- **"The Biology of Cancer" by Robert A. Weinberg:** An authoritative resource that offers a deep dive into the molecular and cellular basis of cancer. Ideal for readers keen on understanding cancer from a biological standpoint.

  - Publisher: Garland Science

- **"The Emperor of All Maladies: A Biography of Cancer" by Siddhartha Mukherjee:** A Pulitzer Prize-winning title, this book chronicles the history of cancer from its first documentation to the latest research, woven with compelling patient stories.

  - Publisher: Scribner

- **"Radical Remission: Surviving Cancer Against All Odds" by Kelly A. Turner, Ph.D.:** This book explores cases where people have defied medical expectations to recover from advanced-stage cancers, identifying common factors that may play a role in their recovery.

  - Publisher: HarperOne

## 2. Prevention and Lifestyle

- **"Anticancer: A New Way of Life" by Dr. David Servan-Schreiber:** Drawing from his own experience with brain cancer, Dr. Servan-Schreiber discusses foods, activities, and mental practices that can help reduce cancer risk and support treatment.

  - Publisher: Penguin Group

- **"The China Study: The Most Comprehensive Study of Nutrition Ever Conducted" by T. Colin Campbell and Thomas M. Campbell II:** A groundbreaking study that links nutrition to cancer, advocating for a whole-food, plant-based diet.

  - Publisher: BenBella Books

## 3. Personal Experiences and Memoirs

- **"When Breath Becomes Air" by Paul Kalanithi:** A neurosurgeon diagnosed with stage IV lung cancer recounts his journey from doctor to patient, exploring life, death, and purpose.

  - Publisher: Random House

- **"The Bright Hour: A Memoir of Living and Dying" by Nina Riggs:** A poignant account of a woman diagnosed with terminal breast cancer, reflecting on motherhood, marriage, and the beauty in everyday moments.

  - Publisher: Simon & Schuster

## 4. Support and Caregiving

- **"Help Me Live: 20 Things People with Cancer Want You to Know" by Lori Hope:** A valuable guide for friends and relatives of cancer patients, offering insights into the emotional landscape of those living with the disease.

  - Publisher: Celestial Arts

- **"The Human Side of Cancer: Living with Hope, Coping with Uncertainty" by Jimmie C. Holland M.D. and Sheldon Lewis:** An exploration of the emotional and psychological challenges faced by cancer patients and their loved ones.

  - Publisher: HarperCollins Publishers

## 5. Children and Cancer

- "Childhood Cancer: A Parent's Guide to Solid Tumor Cancers" by Anne Spurgeon and Nancy Keene:

An informative guide for parents of children diagnosed with cancer, offering medical insights, caregiving advice, and real-life stories.

  - Publisher: Childhood Cancer Guides

## 6. Genetics and Cancer

- "The Family Gene: A Mission to Turn My Deadly Inheritance into a Hopeful Future" by Joselin Linder:

A personal journey through the world of genetics, family history, and the quest to understand and combat a rare genetic mutation.

  - Publisher: Ecco

## In Conclusion

The complexity of cancer means that every person's experience and understanding will differ. These recommended readings offer a broad range of perspectives and information, catering to various needs and interests. Whether you're a patient, caregiver, medical professional, or someone keen to understand more, there's likely a book on this list for you.

# Appendix C: Recipe Ideas for a Cancer-Preventing Diet

Eating a well-balanced diet rich in whole foods can play a pivotal role in cancer prevention. Here are some tasty and nourishing recipes that incorporate cancer-fighting ingredients, keeping both your palate and cells happy. Remember, variety is key, so rotate these ideas and experiment with different whole foods.

## 1. Berry Bliss Smoothie

### Ingredients:

- 1 cup mixed berries (blueberries, raspberries, strawberries)
- 1 banana
- 1 cup spinach
- 1 tablespoon chia seeds
- 1 cup almond milk or water

### Instructions:

6. Combine all ingredients in a blender.

7. Blend until smooth.

8. Pour into a glass and enjoy.

*Note:* Berries are rich in antioxidants and vitamins, while spinach adds a dose of greens, and chia seeds provide fiber.

## 2. Turmeric Lentil Soup

### Ingredients:

- 1 cup lentils, rinsed

- 1 onion, chopped
- 2 carrots, diced
- 2 celery stalks, diced
- 3 garlic cloves, minced
- 1 teaspoon turmeric powder
- 1 teaspoon cumin powder
- 6 cups vegetable broth
- Salt and pepper to taste
- Olive oil for sautéing
- Fresh coriander for garnish

**Instructions:**

1. In a large pot, heat olive oil over medium heat.

2. Sauté onions until translucent. Add garlic, carrots, and celery and cook for another 5 minutes.

3. Stir in turmeric and cumin.

4. Add lentils and vegetable broth. Bring to a boil.

5. Lower the heat and simmer until lentils are tender.

6. Season with salt and pepper.

7. Garnish with fresh coriander before serving.

*Note:* Turmeric contains curcumin, known for its anti-inflammatory properties. Lentils are rich in fiber and protein.

## 3. Broccoli and Walnut Stir-Fry

**Ingredients:**

- 2 cups broccoli florets
- 1 cup bell peppers, sliced
- 1/2 cup walnuts
- 2 tablespoons low-sodium soy sauce

- 1 tablespoon olive oil
- 2 garlic cloves, minced
- 1 teaspoon ginger, minced

**Instructions:**

1. In a pan, heat olive oil over medium heat.

2. Add garlic and ginger and sauté until fragrant.

3. Add broccoli florets and bell peppers. Stir-fry for 5-7 minutes.

4. Stir in walnuts and soy sauce. Cook for another 2 minutes.

5. Serve with brown rice or quinoa.

*Note:* Broccoli is a cruciferous vegetable known for its cancer-fighting properties, and walnuts provide omega-3 fatty acids.

## 4. Omega-packed Salmon Salad

**Ingredients:**

- 1 salmon fillet
- 1 tablespoon olive oil
- Mixed salad greens (spinach, kale, arugula)
- 1/2 avocado, sliced
- 1/4 cup cherry tomatoes, halved
- 1/4 cup cucumber, sliced
- Lemon vinaigrette (juice of 1 lemon, 3 tablespoons olive oil, salt, and pepper whisked together)

**Instructions:**

1. Rub salmon with olive oil, salt, and pepper.

2. Grill or pan-sear salmon for about 4 minutes on each side or until cooked to your liking.

3. On a plate, lay out mixed greens and top with avocado, cherry

tomatoes, and cucumber.

4. Place cooked salmon on top.

5. Drizzle with lemon vinaigrette and serve.

*Note:* Salmon is an excellent source of omega-3 fatty acids, which have anti-inflammatory benefits.

When crafting your meals, remember the importance of colorful plates, whole foods, and unprocessed ingredients. The recipes mentioned here are just starting points; let them inspire you to discover more delicious, health-promoting dishes!

# Appendix D: Glossary of Terms

Below is a glossary of key terms used throughout this book. Familiarizing yourself with these terms can provide a deeper understanding of the content and concepts discussed.

## 1. Antioxidants

Compounds found in food that prevent or delay damage to cells caused by free radicals. They are abundant in fruits, vegetables, and other plant-based foods.

## 2. Benign

Refers to a condition, tumor, or growth that is not cancerous. It doesn't invade nearby tissues or spread to other parts of the body.

## 3. Carcinogen

A substance or agent that can cause cells to become cancerous by altering their genetic structure, leading to the formation of tumors.

## 4. DNA

Deoxyribonucleic acid, the molecules inside cells that carry genetic information and pass it from one generation to the next.

## 5. Epigenetics

The study of changes in gene activity that do not involve alterations to the underlying DNA sequence. These changes can affect an individual's risk of developing certain diseases, including cancer.

## 6. Free Radicals

Unstable molecules that can damage the cells in your body. They can be produced by external sources (like tobacco smoke) or naturally within our bodies as a byproduct of metabolism.

## 7. Genomics

The study of all of a person's genes (the genome) and their interactions with each other and the environment.

## 8. Holistic

Considering the whole person, including physical, mental, emotional, and spiritual aspects, rather than focusing on specific parts or symptoms.

## 9. Immune System

The body's defense system against infections and diseases, including cancer.

## 10. Malignant

Refers to the growth of cancer cells that are not encapsulated and can invade neighboring tissues or spread to other parts of the body.

## 11. Metastasis

The spread of cancer from its primary site to other parts of the body. When cancer cells metastasize, they break away from the original tumor, travel through the bloodstream or lymph system, and form a new tumor in other tissues or organs.

## 12. Oncology

The branch of medicine that deals with the prevention, diagnosis, treatment, and study of cancer.

## 13. Phytochemicals

Compounds found in plants that can help prevent chronic diseases such as cancer. They give fruits, vegetables, grains, and legumes their color, flavor, and disease resistance.

## 14. Radiation

Energy in the form of particles or waves, such as x-rays or gamma rays. Radiation can be used at high doses to treat cancer and at low doses for imaging studies, like x-rays or CT scans.

## 15. Risk Factor

Anything that may increase a person's chance of developing a disease, including cancer. Risk factors can include behaviors, substances, genes, age, gender, and more.

## 16. Tumor

An abnormal mass of tissue that may be benign (not cancer) or malignant (cancer). Tumors can grow and interfere with the digestive, nervous, and circulatory systems, and they can release hormones that alter body function.

## 17. UV (Ultraviolet) Radiation

A type of energy produced by the sun and some artificial sources, such as tanning beds. UV radiation can damage the skin and lead to skin cancer.

## 18. Wellness

A holistic approach to health that encompasses physical, mental, and social well-being, not merely the absence of disease.

This glossary offers concise definitions of terms frequently encountered in the context of cancer prevention and overall health. Readers are encouraged to seek more in-depth explanations and resources when further clarity is needed.

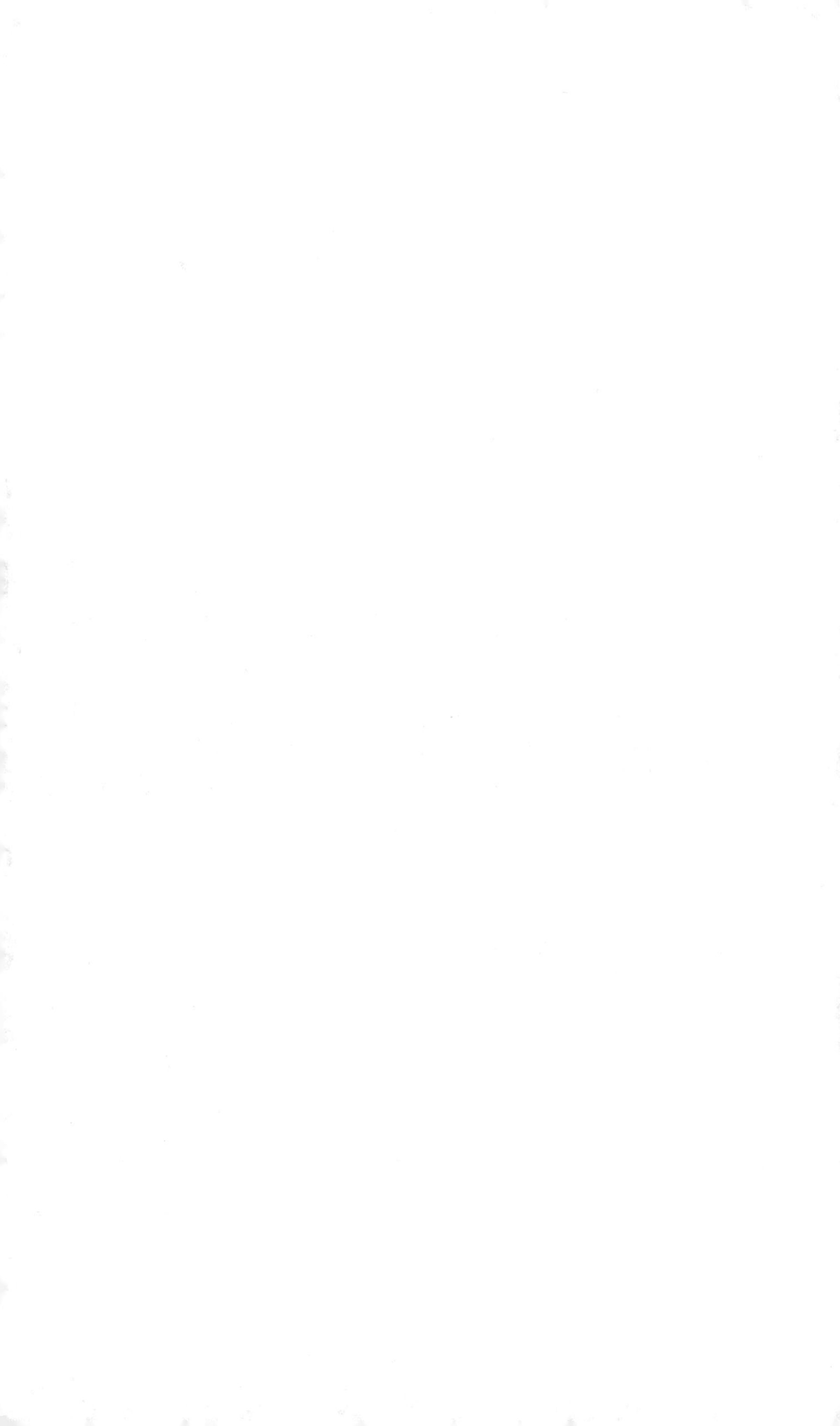

www.ingramcontent.com/pod-product-compliance
Lightning Source LLC
Chambersburg PA
CBHW070952260726
48661CB00003B/1239